Confidence

Hallmarks

Altruism

Romance

Manners

C.H.A.R.M.

How to Make Your World More Beautiful

PRINCESS JULIA KAROLYI

CSP

CONTINENTAL SHELF PUBLISHING, LLC
Savannah, GA
CSPBooks.com

Copyright © 2009 Julia Karolyi

All rights reserved under International and Pan-American Copyright Conventions. No part of this book may be reproduced in any form or by any means, electronic or mechanical, including photocopying, recording by any information storage and retrieval system without written permission by the publisher, except for quotations or excerpts used in reviews or critical articles. For permissions, contact:

Continental Shelf Publishing, LLC • 4602 Sussex Place • Savannah, GA 31405 • www.CSPBooks.com

Photographs by Adam Koenig, courtesy of the author. Make-up and hair styling by Ashley Edwards.

Library of Congress Cataloging-in-Publication Data
Karolyi, Julia.
  C.H.A.R.M. : how to make your world more beautiful / by Princess Julia Karolyi.
     p. cm.
  ISBN 978-0-9822583-1-6 (pbk. : alk. paper)
  1. Charm. 2. Etiquette for women. 3. Beauty, Personal. I. Title. II. Title: Charm.
  BJ1610.K35 2009
  646.7--dc22
                               2009038175

Summary: "Exiled princess and entrepreneur delivers a roadmap to everyday elegance, from stationery to fashion, mixed with strategies on diet, wealth, power. Using the acronym CHARM to illustrate Confidence, Hallmarks, Altruism, Romance and Manners she creates a 21st century twist on old-fashioned charm for greater happiness in love, life, and work."--Provided by publisher

Continental Shelf Publishing books are available at special quantity discounts for premiums, sales promotions, or use in corporate and community training programs. For more information, please contact: Sales@CSPBooks.com

Printed in Canada
First Edition, May 2010

Dedication

For my mother Dorothy and my grandmother Julia.

Contents

You don't have to be born into royalty to give yourself – and others – the royal treatment. Find out how this book will help you CHARM the pants – perfectly tailored and pressed, of course – off of everyone around you as you embark on your mission to make the world a kinder, more beautiful place.

*C*onfidence is CHARMing

Being CHARMing means being good to other people, and you can't do that without first feeling good about yourself – being confident. Feeling beautiful inside and out is a sure way to gain that confidence.

Unveil your true beauty from the inside out with radiance, positive attitude, and a little make-up. Learn beauty secrets that don't come out of a jar (and some that do!).

Why it's not the jiggle as you wiggle but the snap in your step. Ditch the drastic diets and adopt attitudes and habits that will help you stay happy and healthy at any size.

If you want to be CHARMing at any age, then this chapter's got your number! Learn how confidence can grow as you gracefully get up in years.

Hallmarks are CHARMing

Find what makes you unique and play it up! Build a personal brand with a consistent style, image, and attitude. Like greeting cards that send a positive message, your hallmarks – your unique characteristics – tell the world what a CHARMing person you are.

Altruism is CHARMing

It takes a village to be CHARMing. Showing respect for others and being generous in your community are the surprising keys to the city of CHARM.

Romance is CHARMing

Whether you're single and searching or single and satisfied, whether you're attached and happy or attached and antsy, this section's for you. It's all about how romance can and should be a part of everyone's CHARMed lives.

Manners are CHARMing

How we can all serve as models of civility and courtesy in this world by minding our manners.

Foreword

CHARM lays the foundation for a women's revolution unlike anything we have seen before. In the search for equality in the home and workplace, we lost something along the way and Princess Julia Karoly is here to remind us that it is never too late to bring charm—CHARM— back into vogue. Princess Julia has taken her expertise gleaned from years of working within the high-end cosmetic industry and laced it with the childhood training she received at the foot of her grandmother, a member of the exiled royal family of Hungary, to create a one of a kind book that will appeal to women of all ages. Throughout its pages she delivers a personal plan of action to make charm relevant again and provides supportive resources to augment her plan.

Princess Julia's positive style of communication spiced with Southern wit is just the cure for what ails many women who are pressured to do it all in order to have it all. Her message about CHARM is the counterpoint to the endless barrage of ads that dictate youth and beauty as the only assets one must have to be accepted in 21st century society. I especially enjoy the fact that her action plans carry readers through each phase of the aging process with grace and elegance just the way Julia's grandmother taught her, with easily attainable examples of style and sophistication.

CHARM is a must read for every woman.

—Dr. Deborah A. Forrest, Registered Clinical Psychologist

Author, *Symphony of Spirits: Encounters With the Spiritual Dimension of Alzheimer's*

Introduction

The Real Princess Diaries

What does it mean to be a modern day princess? Well, you've come to the right place to find out. I may not live in a castle, and I may not have to cross a moat every time I head out to the grocery store for paper towels, but I was born into a royal family and am very proud of my heritage. (I have been known to take the trash out in a tiara every now and then, if only to keep the neighbors on their toes!) I take it seriously, not because I am better than anyone else. That's not it at all! No, what I take from my heritage is a sense of how to live a full and rewarding life--regardless of wealth-- and how my behavior can serve as a positive model for others and can have a beneficial impact on society.

Partly by nature, partly by nurture, I have made beauty, style, elegance, sophistication, and, most importantly, caring for others, my mission in life.

Simply put, I aim to be charming and to make charm contagious. I am on a mission to make the world a more charming place – a kinder, more courteous, more elegant, more caring place one person at a time, starting with myself. Being charming isn't just about how we look on the outside or old-fashioned feminine wiles.

My kind of charm, the kind I want to share with you in this book, is something altogether new and different. It's not so much charm as it is C.H.A.R.M., or as I like to call it CHARM.

CHARM: A MODERN DAY PRINCESS' TAKE ON MODERN DAY CHARM

Our world has gotten uglier on so many levels, and I'm not talking about bad haircuts, wrinkles, and the wrong lipstick colors. Okay, truth be told, those things bug me, too. But, what I mean when I say the world is uglier is that people are not as caring, courteous, and respectful as they could be, should be, would be if CHARM were their motto.

What is CHARM, as opposed to charm? It's Confidence, Hallmarks, Altruism, Romance, and Manners. The five major sections of this book are organized around these five concepts, but for now let me give you a sneak preview – after all, I'm determined to give you the royal treatment here! So, let's look at what those mean:

♛ Confidence

Feeling good about yourself and being comfortable in your own skin are the first steps toward being CHARMing. You have to like yourself on the inside – your positive attitude and outlook on life– and like yourself on the outside – your beautiful, healthy radiance, whether you were blessed with movie star good looks or the proverbial face only a mother could love. When you feel good from the inside out, yours is a confidence that is truly beautiful and can spread to others.

♛ Hallmarks

You don't have to act like me to be CHARMing. You don't have to act like your neighbor, your favorite supermodel, actress, dignitary, politician, musician, or, for that matter, your favorite princess. You just have to be yourself – a more confident, caring, mannerly self, that is! Your hallmarks are your calling card to the world – your signature style and unique characteristics that people associate with you. The key is that they be *your* hallmarks, not characteristics you've conjured up to be someone or something you're not. Honesty and a clear understanding of who you are make up your hallmarks.

♛ Altruism

The A in CHARM stands for altruism: making the world a better place. An essential element to leading a CHARMed life is family and community work. It is only through caring for others that we take care of the best part of ourselves: our spirit.

♛ Romance

What would CHARM be without a little romance? It's not all about self-esteem and community service and etiquette. There's got to be a spark, too! The romance section of this book helps you find and keep the love you desire, and you might be surprised to learn that loving yourself is the best place to begin.

♛ Manners

The Manners section of this book includes chapters on social, business, travel, and family etiquette. Being CHARMing isn't something you do in just one area of your life. You don't turn it on for the people you want to impress at a party, then come home and be nasty to your family. You don't mind your Ps and Qs at the office then forget manners just because fellow passengers on a flight are strangers you may never see again. Acting with courtesy, politeness, and respect occurs in every corner of your life and every corner of the world if you want to be a bonafide CHARM ambassador.

WHEN DID CHARM GO ON VACATION?

I have been called a "CHARM detective" and, ladies, the clues are getting harder and harder to find these days. Everywhere I go, I'm on the lookout for respect, grace and manners, and I haven't found a single charming clue in weeks!

On the road, people use their middle fingers more often than their turn signals. At work, it's more "What have you done for me lately?" than "What can I do for you?" In stores and restaurants, it takes an act of Congress to get a smile with your service. Even at home, we're often ruder to our own families than we are to total strangers. When did CHARM go on vacation?

I began working for the Revlon Company as a counter girl at the tender age of 16 – the first company hire ever under the age of 21. After Revlon came stints at Clinique, Elizabeth Arden, and Dior. And after that? My own cosmetics company, of course! It's called Beautage® and I'm proud to say it's based in Atlanta, home of southern hospitality.

CHARM is back in vogue and you, dear reader, are among the trendsetters. From now on consider me your lobbyist for loveliness in every nook and cranny of your life. And in this book, no corner of your life is going to go un-CHARMed. Every day, in every way, you're going to be more CHARMing. Your friends and associates are going to notice how much better you look, how much attention you get and, most importantly of all, how self-confident and caring you are.

What's In It For You?

CHARM isn't something you put on when you walk out the door, like a raincoat or Easter hat. CHARM is the daily fuel that drives our success.

♛ More Referrals

When you have CHARM, people notice; the *right* people: the people you want to do business with and make money with. CHARM is the ultimate talent and the ultimate recommendation. Whatever you want more of in the business world, CHARM is the inside track to get it.

♛ Better Social Life

I have a busy social calendar, and it's not because of my bundt cake! People feel good when they're around me, for two good reasons: First, I work hard at making others feel good but, secondly and more importantly, I feel good doing it. And that draws people to me, just like it will draw people to you.

♛ More Business

If you think running a cosmetics company is easy, think again. (Or better yet, try it yourself!) But I have persevered in my business mainly because I chose to do what I enjoy– and what I *love* being *good* at. It's easy to be CHARMing when you're happy about the path your life has taken, and it should come as no surprise that others will want to join you in your journey.

♛ More Bliss

CHARM makes us happy. Why? Because when you're CHARMing, you're running on all cylinders. Your home life's in order, your health, your wealth and well-being are all chugging along as they should. The more CHARMing you are, the happier you are.

♛ More of an Impact

When we are CHARMing, we make more of a positive impact on the world. I'm not saying that you're going to bring about world peace or find a cure for cancer just by being CHARMing. But, you can make a difference by projecting a confident, graceful, respectful air as you work to make the world a better place, whether in your community or around the globe. CHARM is powerful.

A Pure Injection of Charm

Nowhere in this book do I say that CHARM depends on how good-looking you are, or your weight, or age, or race, or sex, or height, or income. That's because none of those things matters when it comes to true CHARM. The best kind of CHARM comes from within. But for CHARM to work its undeniable magic, we have to let it out into the world and share it. Because the one thing about CHARM is that the more you share it, the more CHARMing others become. It's downright contagious, and that's why it's so important for those of us who care about this world to enlist in the CHARMing army now. The sooner we become CHARMing, the sooner all of our friends, family, neighbors, co-workers, and social circle will become CHARMing; it starts with us.

Charm spreads from you to your partner to your family to your friends to your neighbors to your coworkers and to everyone you meet. We're not just making ourselves more beautiful, ladies; we're making history! So let's start spreading a "CHARM virus," shall we? All it takes is one pure injection of equal parts style, empathy and sophistication. And you're about to get a full dose in this book!

You don't have to be born a princess to feel like royalty or to give others the royal treatment! Enjoy!

Love,

Julia

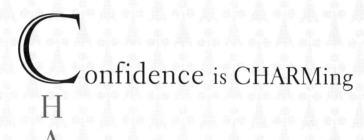

Confidence is CHARMing

Confidence is CHARMing

"Regardless of how you feel inside, always try to look like a winner. Even if you are behind, a sustained look of control and confidence can give you a mental edge that results in victory."

Diane Arbus

Before you can CHARM others, you have to CHARM yourself. You have to feel good about who you are, and then you can help other people feel good about themselves. Without confidence in yourself – believing that you are beautiful inside and out – there will be limits on how CHARMing you can be.

If you already consider yourself to be a confident person, the chapters in this section will help you bump up your self-asssurance. But, if you're like most of us, your confidence wavers day to day, or with each new challenge. As our physical beauty fades, as our weight fluctuates, and good hair days come and go, our confidence can wax and wane.

We may look for more efficient make-up, finer clothes, or the latest anti-aging secrets as solutions to our confidence crashes. While those things can help, they address only part of the issue: outer beauty. What about our inner beauty? What role does it play?

The only certain thing in this life is Uncertainty; conditions change, especially in the physical sense. We have a general sense of dissatisfaction with ourselves. Physical features are impermanent, the constant pursuit of perfection is pointless. Measuring up to the impossible standards set by the fashion industry and flaunted on the red carpet can be withering. But when I think of the truly beautiful women I have known, they all share one thing in common–regardless of their physical attributes: they shine from within, and with a light that does not fade with time, fad or fashion.

Our attitude and disposition play a huge role in our confidence level. The more positive we are, the more we truly respect and care for ourselves and all other human beings, the more CHARMing we are.

So, in these first three chapters, you will find some practical tips on make-up, clothing, weight loss, and aging with grace and charm, but what I really want you to learn is that it's what's inside you that counts most. That's where confidence and the first step in being CHARMing comes from!

Chapter 1

Princess Julia on Beauty

"Zest is the secret of all beauty. There is no beauty that is attractive without zest."

Christian Dior

Most of my professional life has been about beauty. As a young make-up stylist for major cosmetics companies in the early years of my career I helped women be more beautiful with just the right brush stroke here and touch of color there. Later, as I progressed in sales and management roles for those big companies, I marketed beauty, which often came at a high price tag. Lately, as developer of my own skincare line, I've learned the science of beauty – how the ingredients that go into the products we put on our skin can make us more beautiful, and not always necessarily at a high price.

Beauty has become a commodity. We think that with just the right cosmetics or just the right hair style, clothing, or height of heel on our shoe, we can buy beauty. Goodness knows enough people want to sell it to us! But is beauty something we can buy? Of course, not. Sure, we can enhance our beauty – outer beauty, that is – with make-up and haircuts that play up our best features, and with clothes that hide our flaws and accentuate our positives. And if we have lots of money to spend in the beauty and fashion worlds, we can do a lot of enhancing – maybe even the surgical kind!

But, you and I know deep down that beauty can't be bought or sold. It's easy to forget this. After all, I have dedicated my career to the pursuit of beauty, trying to help women achieve it and figuring out how to make myself look as good as I possibly can. Nothing wrong with that! But, it seems the more years I spend in the world of "manufactured beauty," the more I learn that beauty does not come out of a jar or our closets.

Beauty through the Ages – Our Ages

Like CHARM itself, beauty is a sum of many parts. To call someone beautiful is a compliment, of course, but what exactly are we complimenting? Her figure, her dress, her makeup, her nose, her style, her grace? Depending on where you are in life, you hear the word "beauty" and think of a variety of different things – all of which mean beautiful to you.

In our youth, beauty means clear skin, straight teeth, and very cherry lip gloss, which we apply liberally in our fuzzy pink locker mirrors. In our late teens and early adult years beauty often comes in terms of size: size 6 is beautiful and anything else is, well, anything but.

As we get older and the unrealistic expectations of youth get harder and harder to maintain, we turn our attention to other forms of beauty – maybe a gorgeous tan, shimmering hair, full lips, or bigger breasts.

Even later, beauty can be found in the glow of pregnancy or the radiance of childbirth. Still later we consider the absence of wrinkles or gray hair beautiful, and later still we welcome these additions to our aging beauty as signs that we're still alive and vital – a beautiful thing indeed. Beauty, then, isn't just in the eye of the beholder but in the beholder's age as well.

Beauty Is As Beauty Does

I have a girlfriend who is absolutely gorgeous and sexy; she's a curvy size 16. I have another friend who always looks divine and statuesque; she stands 5'2".

One of my most beautiful friends hates her red hair and freckles, another won't wear open-toed sandals because she's afraid to show her less than perfect toes. And one more hasn't been swimming in years because, in her words, "I can't find a bathing suit with a good enough girdle!" Despite all their major differences, what do all these women have in common? One thing: they are Beautiful with a capital "B," but they aren't Confident with a capital "C."

I had friends over for dinner the other night and as I was showing them around the house, one of them picked up an old photograph of me and said, "Julia, you look so beautiful in this picture!" I didn't think much of it at the time – I think I smelled my salmon burning! – but later I looked at the picture and thought, "You know what; he was right – I *did* look pretty good in that picture." Thing was, I hadn't looked at that photo in years and, what's more, I remember when the picture was taken and I had thought I was too this, too that, not enough this, and way not enough that.

I think beauty is like that. How many pictures did we take last year that won't really feel "beautiful" to us until a few more years from now? How many outfits did we not wear because they were too tight, too big, or even just right – but we didn't feel beautiful enough to do them justice? How many invitations did we turn down, picnics did we avoid, or beach houses did we not rent because we didn't quite feel beautiful enough?

But I keep coming back to that picture and thinking, "I looked good then and didn't even know it. What does that say about how I look today?" Fortunately, in my line of work, I can't run from how I look. I'm constantly doing photo shoots for new press kits or brochures or beauty lines and it's hard to avoid looking at yourself when a photographer is handing you a glossy sheet of photos and saying, "Pick one for the back cover!"

Accentuate the Positive

The thing I've learned to do along the way is look at myself objectively; as other people might. It's a good exercise because it makes you realize that, hey, you know what: my nose isn't quite as big as I thought and my ears aren't as small. My hair is okay, and my skin is pretty good, and I like the eyes, and, okay, maybe I'm not so hideous after all.

Then, too, it forces you to find your own flaws. I know my forehead can get shiny in photos so I make sure to handle that and I've learned just what eye shadow colors accent my eyes and

Princess Julia's
CHARM Tip #1

I bet you never – okay, hardly ever – skip a morning or evening when it comes to moisturizing your face, but what about your neck and chest? For beauty longevity, don't forget that the skin on your neck and chest is also vulnerable to sun and environmental toxins and needs to be nourished with a quality moisturizer.

which detract. So what I'm saying is that if you really want to feel beautiful, you've got to face your strengths and weaknesses and address each one accordingly.

For instance, if you have long legs, play them up. Accentuate with just the right size heels and the right length skirt or shorts. Know what looks good and keep doing that. If people have always admired your high cheekbones and lustrous eyes, get a makeover to accentuate those very assets and learn how to do it yourself.

Likewise, if you're not so fond of your hips, experiment with clothes, fabrics, or designers until you find a few that accentuate them rather than objectify them. If your height has always bothered you learn ways to appear taller through sensible heels and certain cuts of clothes that spread your figure out rather than smash it down.

There are many ways to accentuate the positive and blur the negative, if only you'll address each one in kind and take a good, honest look at what you like – and don't like – about how you look. The more familiar with yourself you become, the more beautiful you become.

The Black Hole of Beauty

The thing about beauty is that we always want more. Even if we reach our ideal weight we still can't feel "beautiful" because there's always just one more pound – or two or three or ten – to go. If we get just the right haircut, oh well, it's always too short or too long to us. If we're tall we want to be just a tad not so Amazonian and if we're short we'd love desperately to be an Amazon – and then some!

Princess Julia's Favorite Books on Beauty

Beyond the Body! Developing Inner Beauty by Linda Ellis Eastman (Professional Woman Publishing).

Making Faces by Kevyn Aucoin (Little, Brown & Company).

Staging Your Comeback: A Complete Beauty Revival for Women Over 45 by Christopher Hopkins (HCI).

YOU: Being Beautiful: The Owner's Manual to Inner and Outer Beauty by Michael F. Roizen and Mehmet C. Oz (Free Press).

In our minds, perfection is always defined by things out of our control, like good genes, aging well, a perfect metabolism. Beauty is the finish line no one ever crosses because the definition of beauty is always changing. So if it's ever-changing, what can you do to feel beautiful? I'm glad you asked because, after all, as the owner of a cosmetics company, beauty is my stock and trade.

The Five Qualities of Beauty

What, no makeup tips? No fitness advice? No secret to 30-second abs or 20-minute thighs? That's right; this chapter is about *real* beauty, not a quick fix. Now, more than ever we have the power to make changes in our favor. And like real CHARM, genuine beauty is a multi-faceted diva based on what I've identified as five major qualities:

✳ Style

Much has been said about style but what, really, *is* style? For me, style is your default setting; it's how you look, dress, act, talk, and walk every single day – not just when other people are looking. It's how people think of you when you're not around; the general impression you leave when you get up and walk out of a room. We all know women whose style is glamorous, women who are sexy, women who are frumpy, and women who are trashy. Glamorous, sexy, frumpy, trashy; these are all generic descriptions for a default style that one wears like a sign on their forehead.

The great thing about style is that it's personal to you and, if done right, *any* style can be beautiful. After all, there are a great many women who manage to pull "trashy" off with such enthusiasm, innocence, fun, and aplomb that what might look tacky or tasteless on someone else actually works for them. Pamela Anderson fits into this category. Say what you want, but her skimpy outfits and questionable taste really do seem to work for her. Trust me, that's a compliment! Even frumpy can "fit" if you own that style and make it your own. Think Annie Hall or Maude, and you'll get a general idea of where I'm going with this. My point is, whatever your style, it can be beautiful if you make it your own and positively enjoy it.

❋ Grace

Grace is the art of staying calm – and looking serene – even when the world is dissolving around you. Think of the world's most classically beautiful, elegant, and simply gorgeous women – Audrey Hepburn, Sophia Loren, Lauren Bacall, Lena Horne, Grace Kelly – and one word comes to mind: grace. How is grace beauty? The same way wearing just enough foundation is the base for a perfectly made-up face, the same way gauging just the right dress to wear to the cocktail party allows your figure to really shine, and the same way pulling your hair back can show off your elegant forehead, grace is the underpinning of beauty, allowing you to be your most beautiful self. Being graceful might not make you beautiful, in and of itself, but with grace, beauty comes more naturally, more easily than without it.

✳ Health

I don't care what those skinny supermodels from Manhattan say, you can't be beautiful if you're not healthy. Like style and grace before it, health is an undercurrent of authentic beauty. It's the glow of a healthy woman that makes her truly attractive. It's the spring in her step, bounce in her walk, curve of her hips, or fullness of her face. When you're too much of anything – too heavy, too thin, too well-muscled, not muscled enough – you're not quite healthy. Health has been said to be a balance of all things – sweet and sour, heavy and thin, hot and cold, happy and sad. Somewhere in the middle we achieve a healthy balance that creates a beauty no makeup can cover, no blouse can conceal, and no mirror can deny. When women come to me for tips, I often notice that their priorities are out of whack. "Seek health before beauty," I always say, "and one will surely follow the other."

✳ Well-being

Well-being is not quite the same thing as health because like makeup, skin, hair, or figure, health is only one part of well-being. Like style, well-being is that big thing that so many other little things go into creating; it's the sum of the parts, not a part in and of itself. If style is the default setting for your body, then well-being is the default setting for your mind; it's how you feel 99.9% of the time. It's when you wake up, after lunch, before dinner, reading in bed, as you lay your head down on the pillow. Well-being is that current that flows through your day. If you're unwell, the current is negative and the opposite of what is beautiful. But if you're well, the current is steady, positive, and downright radiant.

❊ Confidence

To me, confidence isn't just one facet or quality of beauty but confidence *is* beauty in and of itself. I don't care what you look like – big teeth, coke-bottle glasses, stringy hair, knobby knees, or pointy nose – if you have confidence you *can* pull it off and, what's more, you *can* be beautiful. Haven't you ever been at a dinner party or a nice restaurant and watched a confident woman walk into the room? I'm not talking the false confidence of youth or the entitlement of money, or even the brash confidence of the movie star or model, but the true inner confidence of someone who has her act together and knows she's beautiful, no matter what modern conventions say. People are attracted to confident people no matter what they look like. I've rarely encountered a pretty CEO, but I've seen a lot of beautiful women executives. What's the difference? Take women like Cathleen Black, president of Hearst Magazine Division, or Shelly Lazaarus, CEO of Ogilvy & Mather, or Meg Whitman, former CEO of eBay. Not classically beautiful women, per se, but strong, confident, and, therefore, beautiful women each in their own way.

You Are So Beautiful... To You!

There is only one person who can decide if you are beautiful, and I think we both know who that is already: YOU! And yet so many of us get caught up in the comparison crunch. We compare ourselves to the most unrealistic and unlikely role models: movie stars, teenagers on reality shows, models, and supermodels; women whose job it is to look good, with all the attentive attendants money can buy: hairstylists, makeup artists, dieticians, nutritionists, personal trainers, personal chefs, personal shoppers, and personal stylists!

I'm as bad as anybody else; it can be fun to check out the gossip rags or flip through fashion magazines at the beauty salon. But the one place we all should be looking for beauty tips is straight in the mirror.

You can chase celebrity fad diets, guaranteed makeup tips from the stars, and supermodel fat flush plans until you're blue in the face, exhausted, and nowhere close to your ideal image of beauty. Or you can look in the mirror, get to know the one

---

Princess Julia's
Pet Peeve #1: Arrogance

I've met A-list actors, CEOs, millionaires, and billionaires, and there are two kinds of each – those who think they're better than everybody else and those who know they're just a stock market crash, bomb movie, or scandal away from washing their own dishes and digging ditches for a living, so they are grateful for everything they have and humbled by their good fortune. But the others – the arrogant ones – what an ugly way they go through life. Arrogance is a huge pet peeve of mine because no one – not the President, not supermodels, not billionaires, or movie stars or maitre d's – is entitled to think that he or she is better than anyone else. Arrogance is so un-CHARMing!

person who really matters and concentrate on honing your style, grace, health, well-being, and confidence until you not only look beautiful but feel beautiful as well. Now that's something worth chasing!

Parting Words on Beauty

In the final analysis, how beautiful you are doesn't so much have to do with how you look but how you feel. Haven't you ever had a morning where everything goes right? Your hair doesn't get that little kink to the left, your mascara goes on without clumping, your lipstick doesn't smudge, your skirt isn't wrinkled, and your blouse hangs just right. You look in the mirror and for one split-second you have no complaints; there is absolutely nothing to find fault with. And as you step out of the house you feel absolutely invincible.

That, ladies, is beauty. That's how beauty is supposed to feel – flawless and perfect and flattering. Now, you may look like a hen in a handbag, a pig in a blanket, or a wolf in sheep's clothing by some people's standards - those standards shouldn't mean a thing to you – but you feel great.

What happens next is up to you. You can continue to feel as beautiful as when you left the house that morning, or you can let the world intrude and convince you that you're not quite so pretty after all. You can compare yourself to the fancy neighbor getting in her car, the sexy secretary when you get to work, the girls in the fashion magazines as you eat lunch, and your flawless boss as you get ready to leave work. But know this: Each time you do the comparison crunch your confidence goes down a notch. Don't let that happen!

True beauty takes stock of its imperfections, makes compensations, and moves on to more important aspects of the total woman. All of us have imperfections. Let us resolve to be perfect in our imperfections.

Chapter 2

Princess Julia on
Weight and Dieting

*"I've been on a constant diet for the last two decades.
I've lost a total of 789 pounds. By all accounts, I should
be hanging from a charm bracelet."*

Erma Bombeck

If you're anything like me – if you're anything like 99.9% of women in America today – you've been on as many diets as you have vacations. And, those diets probably last just about as long as a vacation. I was heavy as a child, and then around age sixteen I lost a lot of weight and looked and felt great. The weight stayed off until I was in my mid-thirties. But then I experienced three miscarriages, and the subsequent stress of those tragedies along with my hormonal fluctuations led to another bout of weight gain. I tried high protein diets and working out with weights at the gym with a personal trainer, but it didn't work. I clearly wasn't doing enough cardiovascular exercise to get the pounds off. I was rock hard from the weight training and protein but was not doing enough things to burn fat.

Then, lo and behold, I added cancer to the mix. Yes, a bout with ovarian cancer not only took the obvious toll on my mental and physical health that you would expect, but the synthetic hormone replacement I was treated with after surgery shot my weight up more. Only when I switched to natural hormone replacement, modified my diet to sensible, balanced, and portion-controlled nutrition, and started moving my body, did I lose the weight. I've now kept it off for many years and intend never to go back.

Now, I'm no nutritionist, dietician, physician, or fitness expert, but through my own medical and weight-loss battles and by consulting with the best experts, I've learned what works for me and what seems to work for most people. But let me tell you what doesn't work: diets don't work and the latest fad exercise regimens don't work.

What? You don't believe me? You *still* think diets work? Still think if you eat only peanut butter for 80 days or cabbage and watermelon seeds for two weeks straight that you'll fit in that bikini by the time your timeshare's ready in Miami? All right, fair enough; I didn't want to do this, not so soon in our new relationship, but I guess I'll have to introduce you to three of my friends who also think dieting still works.

Melissa Monday

Melissa Monday is stuck in a time warp. Despite the fact that she's spent nearly 2,000 Mondays on this planet, Melissa *still* believes that Mondays are some magical day when she'll no longer feel hungry at lunch or need anything more than bean sprouts and fat-free dressing for dinner.

"On Monday," she reasons, "I'll have none of the cravings for, say, chocolate-covered cherries or pepperoni pizza like I did all weekend. I'll magically, miraculously and suddenly feel no hunger after 6 p.m. and will wake up revived, refreshed, and ready to jog three miles first thing Monday morning. Until then, of course, sky's the limit!"

So all weekend, Melissa treats herself to whatever she wants. A little drive-thru on the way home from work Friday night, ice cream while she's watching TV, some waffles for breakfast Saturday morning, something gooey and fried while she's having lunch with friends, something hearty and saucy as she and her boyfriend have dinner on date night, plenty of snacks in the midnight movie, a breakfast buffet on Sunday, and whatever the heck she wants the rest of the day!!!

Why? Because come Monday she'll finally start that diet of hers. Which diet? The diet she was going to start last Monday, and the Monday before that, and the first Monday of last year, and the first Monday of her new job, and the first Monday she turned 21. It's the same Monday diet she's wanted to start since she turned 13, and, nearly 27 years later, she's *still* hoping this Monday will be the magic Monday.

Of course, she's forgetting that last Monday was supposed to be magic Monday. And she did actually have some success that Monday. She started the first day of her new week with some eggs and coffee, had a salad for lunch, and, despite the fact that she was starving after the gym, she had only soup and an apple for dinner.

Tuesday morning she felt pretty good, although she got up late and had to have one of those chewy granola bars from the gas station on her way to work, and of course some iced mocha coffee to wash it down with.

And by lunch she was starving so she had a tuna fish sandwich, and she wasn't *going* to eat the chips but she'd already screwed up with the granola bar so why not, and by that afternoon she found herself standing in front of the vending machine with a handful of quarters and pushing buttons like crazy. Four bags of chips later, she slumped over her desk in a manufactured sodium-induced high, greasy fingers and all, looking for her lost will power in that stack of empty bags.

But by then it was too late; Melissa Monday was already looking ahead to next Monday, when she'd start all over again. But this week? Well, she'd already gone and ruined it, so why not enjoy the next five days of freedom before it starts all over again?

Felicity Friday

Felicity Friday is the exact opposite of Melissa Monday; instead of freeing herself from the shackles of her weekday diet she pays penance by starving herself all weekend. Her weakness is the cafeteria and the food court, the cubicle snack drawer, and the drive-thru fast lanes on the way home every day from work. So for five days straight she indulges herself on the way to, at, on break from, and driving home from, work – eating like she's a ninth-grader burning off 4,000-calories a day.

The weekend is when she can stare down her inhibitions and pay the ultimate price for having overindulged all week.

So she endures a Friday night bowl of fruit salad with yogurt before an early bed, then it's up at dawn the next morning for a three-mile run, followed by grapefruit before a trip to the gym, and many bottles of water in between. Later it's a salad for lunch before a power walk around the mall with friends, then maybe a bike ride in the afternoon with her hubby before she talks him into grilling fish on the barby.

Sunday it's another twenty-four hours of Herculean exercise, from the gym to the salad bar and back again, all so she can snag that first glistening donut in the lobby café of her office building first thing Monday morning and start the cycle all over again.

In Felicity Friday's world, you can do whatever you want while you're at work – eat it all, sit it out, skip the gym, and double-up on the fries – as long as you torture yourself every weekend with non-stop calorie counting and heart rate checking.

Jada Gym Bag

The only type of fasting Jada Gym Bag believes in is a steady diet of self-abuse. From her pre-work workout to her evening jog, she is a one-woman fitness machine. No need to watch weight here. She burns more calories than a first grader at a Chuck E. Cheese party – and eats twice as much.

But that's okay. For every burger she runs a mile, for every slice of cheesecake she works her glutes, for every glass of wine she takes a spin class. It's a cause and effect relationship that's been dysfunctional for years, but it works for her – even though she can't figure out why her dress size keeps going up, not down.

This is nothing new for Jada; she's been doing it since high school, when she was a track star and could burn off a three-burger after-school binge with a few quick lopes around the track after everyone else had gone home. But now that she's in her mid-thirties, the miles don't come quite as easy and the burgers stay put – right there on her firm thighs and "generous" backside.

The worst part is, Jada actually used to *enjoy* exercise. A trip to the gym was another excuse to get her endorphin rush, that runner's high was like a real one – addictive and positively thrilling while it lasted and even hours afterward. But now it's the food that gives her the high, and the exercise is merely her punishment.

> *"You have to stay in shape. My grandmother, she started walking five miles a day when she was 60. She's 97 today and we don't know where the hell she is."*
>
> Ellen DeGeneres

Don't Put Your Life On Hold – Let it Off the Hook!

Do my friends Melissa Monday, Felicity Friday, and Jada Gym Bag sound eerily familiar? Maybe they're your friends, too. Maybe they sound a lot like someone you know – or several someones you hang out with every day. Maybe they even sound a lot like you. Maybe you have parts of all three of them in you, depending on the week, the month, or the year, all fighting to get out and derail your healthy lifestyle.

The sad part about my three friends – and everyone else who obsesses constantly about their weight and puts "good and bad" connotations on food and fitness – is that they're forgetting the most joyful part about being a woman: loving our bodies, enjoying feeling good, and being proud of looking good, no matter what our shape or size.

Melissa spends every weekend dreading Monday to the point that no matter what she puts in her mouth she can't actually enjoy it because, in her mind anyway, she'll never be able to have it again. Felicity works her butt off all week only to ramp up and work twice as hard over the weekend paying for sins she didn't commit all week. And Jada? Jada's stuck between a candy wrapper and a hard place; she doesn't enjoy the food because she knows she'll only have to work it off afterward

Princess Julia's
CHARM Tip #2

For a true measure of how healthy or unhealthy your weight is, pay attention to your Body Mass Index (BMI) score, not just the numbers on your scale. The Centers for Disease Control and Prevention website (www.cdc. gov) has a handy BMI calculator. All you need to know is your height and current weight to determine if you're in the normal weight range or if you've got some work to do to get there.

and she doesn't enjoy working out anymore because it's only a means to an end.

What do they all have in common? Simple: their life is inevitably, interminably on hold until they look better, until they are slimmer, until they lose weight, until they can fit in this or put on that.

Life is not meant to be put on hold. I've known women who've starved themselves for years and never cracked a smile. I never want to look like that – absolutely thin but completely unhappy.

If you've got some curves, I say, flaunt them! The best part about beauty – and the easiest part of CHARM – is that it's in the eye of the beholder. So if you're not Twiggy, just find someone who digs Miss Piggy!

Don't Weigh Yourself; W.A.Y. Yourself!

I can still remember my gym teacher telling us girls to weigh ourselves before class and after class, just to see how good an hour of exercise could do a young, growing body. Had this poor woman never heard of water weight? That was no true measure of how much weight we'd lost, only how much water weight we'd sweated off, only to be gained again on our first trip to the water fountain between classes.

You probably know that muscle weighs more than fat. So, if you're active, healthy, and create a body that is firm and muscular – no matter what it looks like – you'll actually weigh more than if you had less muscle.

But isn't muscle supposed to be good for us? Well, sure it is. Muscle helps us recover from injury sooner, cushions our bones, and helps boost our metabolism so we don't hold onto as much fat. So what are we to do? Avoid gaining muscle, even with all of its many health benefits? With so many confusing signals, from misguided gym teachers, to doctors, to scientists, to so-called fitness gurus, to talk show hosts, who to believe? One person: yourself.

Instead of weighing yourself every day, I say do it your W.A.Y.:

✳ Work

Work hard to understand what it is YOU want to look like. Remember to picture yourself kindly – but don't let yourself off the hook either, you've got work to do. If you've tried every diet in the world to no avail, but you can maintain how you currently look by eating reasonably and exercising regularly, why fix what's not broken in the first place? Work at maintaining the balanced lifestyle that affords you this look.

✳ Achieve

Aim to achieve realistic personal goals, not unrealistic ones. Put away the women's magazines, tape measure, and celebrity rags. You know your body better than anyone else; you know what's realistic for you and what isn't. Listen to yourself first and everyone else second (except when medical attention is called for, of course!).

✳ Yes

Yes is a word you can use again. We've said "no" to ourselves for far too long. No carbs, no eating after seven o'clock, no dessert, but we do it anyway. Instead of saying "no" all the time we should just give in and say "yes" – within limits. My grandmother used to say "everything in moderation." So far, it's been the best diet advice anyone's ever given me. If you can't stay within limits, maybe you're "eating in" emotions–look at how you feel every time your reach for a "treat," then decide if you really want to eat or walk around the block! You decide.

Worry Less, Do More

Look, we all know how to diet. We should; we've been doing it all of our lives. But isn't the point of a diet to lose weight and then maintain it? Where is the maintenance phase? How come we never get to *that* part? If all our cabbage patch, coffee grounds, lettuce, and pickle diets worked so well, shouldn't we be a nation of slim people?

I think we need to worry less and just do more. Wouldn't life be so much simpler if food, exercise, diet, and carbs or fat intake didn't rule every minute of every day? It doesn't have to. Not anymore.

We know what works for us for breakfast. Whether it's toast and tea, or bacon and eggs, or cereal and milk, or yogurt and fruit, we know when we've had too much, know when we're too full, or something feels just right.

For me, feeling good about myself starts with eating just enough at each meal but not too much, and doing something physical every day of the week – whether it's a brisk walk around my neighborhood, a formal workout at the gym, or just a morning out walking the dog.

Am I a stick thin model? No, but then I never wanted to be. I've been around long enough to know that it's not the jiggle as you wiggle but the snap in your step that counts when it comes to CHARM. There are plenty of big, bold, beautiful women who not only enjoy a good meal now and then but also enjoy how they look with a little meat on their bones.

A voluptuous Queen Latifah, a juicy Mariah Carey, a lush and lovely Jennifer Lopez, and a powerfully positive America Ferrara – let these be our inspirations over some unrealistically thin model or anorexic actress. I have nothing against how one woman wants herself to look; I have everything against the rest of us thinking we have to look exactly like her to be beautiful.

CHARM isn't just about a number on a scale or a size on the waistband of your favorite linen pants. CHARM is the whole package – how you hold yourself, enjoy life, treat your friends, smile, walk into a room, or dress for the figure you have.

We all know women who are positively tiny and make it their life's mission to stay that way. Have you ever stood next to one at a party? Tried to make conversation as you walk through the buffet line? Or sat next to one on a bus? It's chilling; every word, every syllable, every thought is about food. How to deny themselves, judge you, and impress the world with how great they can look by eating so little.

Where is the CHARM in that? Where is the joy in a good meal? It comes down to this: if you can't do someone the honor of enjoying a piece of cake on their birthday, you may not have learned the art of balance and swaps-- eat a little, diet a little, exercise always. You just can't have it all at the same time. But depriving yourself will only make matters worse. Start by being

Princess Julia's
Favorite Books on Weight and Dieting

Mindful Eating: A Guide to Rediscovering a Healthy and Joyful Relationship with Food by Jan Bays (Shambhala Publishing).

Women, Food and God: An Unexpected Path to Almost Everything by Geneen Roth (Scribner).

Eat This, Not That! Thousands of Simple Food Swaps that Can Save You 10, 20, 30 Pounds--or More! by David Zinczenko and Matt Goulding (Rodale Books).

The End of Overeating: Taking Control of the Insatiable American Appetite by David Kessler (Rodale Books).

French Women Don't Get Fat by Mireille Guiliano (Knopf).

Hungry Girl: Recipes and Survival Strategies for Guilt-Free Eating in the Real World by Lisa Lillien (St. Martin's Griffin).

kind to yourself. Nurture your true needs first, and stop using food as a reward or cover-up for those feelings we don't want to confront. Change is a long process, so stick to it until it's second nature. I want to encourage you on by saying that doctors believe if you stay on a new regimen for as little as two months, your brain incorporates that as your new standard, so it's easier to stick to that new diet or regimen.

Cheat More, Weigh Less

When we go off our diet, we call it cheating, but if we're only cheating ourselves, then I say give me a failing grade but I become accountable to myself. I'm serious about this; life is not meant to be lived on protein and veggies alone. I believe if God had intended for us to be a size zero, She wouldn't have invented coconut pie, lasagna, and sweet tea. But remember *balance*: a little goes a long way, so you don't need to overindulge either.

You can enjoy life and look your best if only you'll give yourself a break! Stop counting calories and start paying attention to your body and your emotions. Eat just a little more slowly so you can listen to your body's signals and, when you're *almost* full, stop eating. Savor each bite carefully, paying attention to the texture of the the food. Play a game of how many different flavors you can find in each bite: the bitter, the sweet, the tart, savory. As you pay more attention to what you're eating, you will find that you will eat more slowly. Forget multitasking: put away the magazine or newspaper, turn off the TV: pay attention to your food, savor and chew! My grandmother used to say: drink your solids and chew your liquids-- I never got that until I started eating ever so slowly. Yes, it really is that simple.

Move more often and enjoy doing it. You don't have to go to a gym to burn calories; clean your house, weed your garden, help a friend move – there are dozens, hundreds of books written on diet and exercise so I'm not going there, but I will say this: when we use words like "good and bad," "off your diet or on," "cheating" or "reward," we're putting too much emotional emphasis on food and not enough on *why we eat when we're not really hungry in the first place.*

Princess Julia's
Pet Peeve #2: Insecurity

It really upsets me to see someone who is insecure, because I know that the only reason they feel down on themselves is that they haven't learned this one simple rule about life: we are all special, unique, and gifted. You are special, and that's nothing to feel insecure about. Whatever it is you do, and maybe you just haven't discovered it yet, that thing you do is unique and exclusive to you. Be proud of it, even if it's something that will never make you a million dollars or movie-star famous. Don't compare yourself to others; that's a lose-lose proposition that can only lead to insecurity and shatter your confidence.

Reach for your running shoes before opening that fridge or that candy bar, brew fresh herbal tea, drink a full glass of water, put out the garbage, occupy yourself until the craving goes away.

Remember that how much we weigh is only part of our overall CHARM. It's maybe one-tenth, or even one-twentieth of the whole package. Being compassionate and generous, being productive and contributing to our workplace or society, sharing a smile and a laugh long and often, feeling confident – these are some of the things that make us CHARMing. When you remember how much else goes into the CHARM equation you'll tend to focus a little less on something miniscule like weight and more on how much else you truly have to offer.

Now, this advice comes with one caveat: I'm not one to support you being any size you want and letting it go at that. Some women can be perfectly healthy at size 20 and have no ill effects, while others can suffer from high blood-pressure and other health problems at a size 14. I want you to *be* healthy as well as *look* healthy. If you can be a big, beautiful, sumptuous large size and the doc gives you a clean bill of health, more power to you. But if you feel unhappy and unhealthy at any size, you need to pay attention to that as well and get proper medical care.

Don't Be On a Diet, Just Be Yourself

The bottom line on diet is that life is a journey, not a destination. Never once have I heard someone say they're at their ideal weight. I love the line in *The Devil Wears Prada* when Emily, the snooty assistant, says, "I'm just one stomach flu away from my goal weight." Isn't that how many of us secretly feel some of the time? But the minute we get close to the finish line, somebody moves it again!

So quit starving yourself and just be yourself. Look at yourself in the mirror – realistically – and love what you see. It may not be perfect, but it's you; for better or worse. If you want to get in better shape or lose weight for health reasons, be my guest. But if you're doing it to impress friends or look like Amy Actress or Melanie Model, well, you've got bigger problems than a few waist sizes, believe you me!

Chapter 3

Princess Julia on
Aging Beautifully

"Age is an issue of mind over matter. If you don't mind, it doesn't matter."

Mark Twain

My Aunt Grace, my mother's sister, owned a beauty salon for nearly forty years and always took care of herself in the same way she took care of her clients. She's retired now and in her early seventies and has aged beautifully. She has always been a fanatic about her skin and hair, not just "putting on her face" and "doing her hair," but keeping them squeaky clean and treating them with care through the use of quality products. But you know what has made her age even more gracefully than that? Her outlook on life. She always has a smile on her face, she is always happy. When she had her salon, clients could count on her to make them feel good with her sunny, entertaining disposition, and she hasn't lost that in retirement. If only I can age as gracefully as my aptly named Aunt Grace!

Age is Not a Four-Letter Word

This is a chapter I couldn't wait to write because, let's face it: I've been working up to it all my life! Aging is a subject on many people's minds these days – particularly the older they get – and yet the minute we hear the word "aging" many of us tense up and get worried.

Aging has become a bad word, something best left unsaid but far from untreated. In fact, we attack aging with a vengeance, as if it is a battle to be won or, at the very least, fought vigorously until the bitter, wrinkly end. The war cry is heard everywhere you listen: "Whatever it takes, however much it costs, whoever we need to consult, we will win this battle!"

The American attitude toward aging seems to be the same as our attitude toward car repair. (Stick with me here!) Instead of regular upkeep and preventive maintenance on our cars, we generally just drive them into the ground and get them fixed when they break down (typically on the side of the road at the worst possible time).

Forget the fact that regular oil changes, tune-ups, alignments, and tire-rotation can save us thousands in repair costs and days spent waiting for the transmission to be rebuilt. We figure if we have a AAA membership we don't have to worry about all that, right?

Well, we tend to treat aging in much the same manner. Why eat right, exercise, quit smoking, and take care of ourselves throughout our lives when we can do whatever we want for fifty, sixty, or seventy years, and, at the first signs of sagging, drooping, puffing, poofing, or wrinkling, we can just go get a few handy procedures done and solve the problem?

Now, I'm not one to come down hard on one side or the other of the plastic surgery issue. I have friends who love it and friends who hate it; I've seen good results and bad. Then again, I run a cosmetics company designed to keep women beautiful throughout their long, healthy lives so I tend to be in favor of "slow and steady" versus "slice and dice." But that's just me.

This chapter is all about aging gracefully whether a little nip and tuck is part of the picture or not. It's about creating a new attitude of acceptance and understanding toward aging so that when it inevitably occurs we are not only better armed to eradicate it but better prepared to deal with it with confidence.

If Age Is Nothing But a Number, Dibs on 18!

Now, I'm as big a fan of clichés as the next gal, but anyone who tells you that "Age is nothing but a number" is, pardon my French, full of it. Have these fools ever had a hot flash, hemorrhoid, or hangnail? How about a cold that lasts two weeks, a donut that takes two months to burn off, or a knee that gets sore sitting down in the pew, let alone kneeling on Sunday morning?

Here's a cliché I can really sink my teeth into: "Aging ain't for sissies!" Among the many joys you'll experience as you age are these gems:

✳ Slower Metabolism

Wasn't it just yesterday when I could down a heaping plate of pasta and it would disappear off my waist and thighs as soon as I laced up my running shoes, let alone hit the pavement for a nice, long jog? These days it takes me longer and longer to get rid of what I eat less and less of. I compare my metabolism to my computer; the older I get, the slower it gets!

❋ Faster Deterioration

Not a day goes by when I don't notice significant changes in this jalopy I call a body. From sore knees, to neck aches, to that dull throbbing in the middle of my back, let's just say my body sometimes feels like it's ready for a trade-in!

❋ Longer Healing Times

My friend broke her arm last summer and I'm still waiting for her to heal. I had a cold last winter and I think I just got over it! Seriously, healing times can not only double as you age but quadruple, and I just don't bounce back the same way I used to. I'm far from housebound, in fact I'm quite energetic, but it's to the point now where my age is forcing me to make difficult choices. For instance, I stay out dancing too late on Friday night, then workout at the gym on Saturday, I might be aching by the time I go for a long walk with the dog and my friends on Sunday. I can't necessarily do it all. These are choices you don't have to make at sixteen.

❋ Less Immunity

Lately I catch everything. While traveling last month I had to check out of my hotel because I could smell the mold in the room the minute I walked in. Call it a "sick sense," but I knew if I stayed there longer than I took to un-sanitize the bathroom I'd come down with a nasty sinus infection the minute I got home. I notice more and more people coughing and sneezing, too, maybe because I'm so paranoid about coming down with something. You think after a lifetime of being among the public exposed to every germ known to humans I'd have the immune system of a cyborg by now, but just the reverse seems true: I'm as vulnerable as a six-day old infant.

Princess Julia's
CHARM Tip #3

Always wear sunglasses! You'll get a triple dose of protection – preserving your eyes' health, preventing brown spots around the eyes, and staving off wrinkles.

How to Age Gracefully

Reading over that last section aging doesn't sound too CHARMing, does it? But that's the thing about aging: it makes you work extra hard to have half the grace you did just a few years ago.

Now, as far as I'm concerned there are really only two ways to age: with class or without. (Guess which one includes spandex.) And, since this is a book called CHARM, I'm talking about the CHARMing way to age, which includes more style and grace and less smoke and mirrors.

Sometimes we learn as much from how not to do something as we do from how to do it, and aging is definitely one of these cases. I mean, it's harder to spot someone who's aging gracefully – which is exactly the point, by the way – than it is someone who is not aging gracefully. (The tube top, hoop earrings and jet black dye job are usually dead giveaways.)

Here are my five tips on how to age gracefully:

❊ DON'T Dress Like Your Daughter

Aging gracefully is all about having a natural progression from year to year. Anything too severe, unsightly, young, or fake is definitely out. I play a little game with my friends when we're ready to go out and one of us is dressing a little too young for my taste. It's called "One of these things is not like the other." You can play it, too. Simply look in the mirror and try to spot what doesn't go with everything else you're wearing. Be it sparkly strawberry milkshake lipstick, a B-52s button on your lapel, or a bright pink dolphin ankle bracelet poking out from beneath your pleated slacks, if it doesn't fit, it ain't legit.

❊ More is NOT Less

My philosophy is the older I get, the fewer bangles, bows, bells and whistles I need to draw attention to that fact. More is NOT less but less is definitely more. The good thing about aging is that it lets us all get back to the basics -- basic hairstyles that flatter us, basic colors that suit us, and basic wardrobe elements and accessories that complement our graceful progress through this life.

❊ Severity DOES NOT Equal Youth

Youth equals fullness. If you look at young people, what is remarkable, radiant, and attractive about them is the fullness, the roundness of their features. That "glow" is not from a jar or scalpel but from their supple, full, and radiant skin tone. Don't be afraid to keep a little excess weight on as you age. I consider it a small insurance policy against the too-thin, too-tight look so many women go for as they fight to reclaim their youth and beauty. And if you *are* getting procedures done, speak with your doctor about creating a natural look that doesn't shock your friends and family the minute you're out of the recovery room.

✳ Plastic Belongs In Your Recycling Bin, Not Your Body

My cosmetic company specializes in producing Beautage™, an effective treatment for all people, men and women, desiring simple usage, non-invasive application, and affordable care for wrinkled or environmentally abused skin. As a make up artist, sales executive, and business owner, I have seen and experienced the importance of first impressions, appearance and positive response to a professional personal appearance. Working for some of the largest and best cosmetic companies in the industry has reinforced in me the absolute necessity for good skincare in order to achieve and maintain youthful, properly hydrated, satin soft skin. Plastic doesn't belong in that equation.

✳ Don't Lie, Deny

Most people would never be rude enough to ask how old a woman is. (At least, not where I'm from.) But if they do, the proper response is not to shave five, ten or fifteen years off of your real age but to tell the truth. Or, if you don't want to reveal your age, then simply deflect the question. If the person you're speaking to insists on continuing this ill-mannered line of conversation, well, they're not very worthy of your CHARM now, are they?

Why Grace and Age Go Hand in Hand

Aging is inevitable; there's just no way to stop it. And those who try the hardest often end up looking the oldest, most severe, most obvious, and least attractive. I'm not saying give in to age entirely; quitting isn't CHARMing.

However, there is a time when you have to concede to the victor and, in this case, age trumps everyone and everything eventually. So, what do you do in the inevitable face of age? Well, where I grew up the Southern style dictates us all to age gracefully and that's good enough for me. Aging gracefully is more than just a clever cliché or turn of phrase. For me, it's a way of life. G.R.A.C.E. stands for:

✳ **Gracious**

Grace is to being gracious what fame is to being famous. In other words, you can't have one without the other. But the best part about being gracious is that it's a synonym for cordial. God, how I love that word! Cordial. Doesn't it just scream grace, class, and charm?

✳ **Restore**

The *worst* things I can say about aging is that it saps us of our energy, our youth, our vitality, and our enthusiasm. It is up to us to be vigilant against signs of aging and actively fight to restore those very things it robs us of.

❋ Aware

The *best* thing I can say about aging is that once we've learned not to worry about every little thing, we are awakened to that which makes life worth living in the first place: family, friends, the satisfaction derived from doing good work, and the joy of simple pleasures. With age comes awareness and a reawakening to our true purpose in life.

❋ Carefree

The best antidote to aging is not so much what we can do physically to reverse it but what we can do mentally to enjoy it. As Mark Twain said of aging, "If you don't mind, it doesn't matter." Have a carefree attitude about your advancing years. Think of all the vibrant, happy, radiant people who are in their 60s, 70s, 80s, and even 90s who live every day as if it were their last and couldn't care less about age; it's just a number. Don't just envy them; emulate them!

❋ Energetic

Energy is the antidote to most of what aging saps from our bodies, our spirits, and our souls. If we can keep vital, in motion and full of energy we can fight aging where it *really* counts: in the mind.

These are your tools, ladies; this is the only ammunition you need to stave off the effects of aging with CHARM, humility and G.R.A.C.E. You don't need expensive procedures, a whole new wardrobe, or someone to convince you that you can reverse aging, stop aging, or even deny aging.

Princess Julia's Favorite Books on Aging Beautifully

The Blue Zones: Lessons for Living Longer From the People Who've Lived the Longest by Dan Buettner (National Geographic).

How Not to Look Old: Fast and Effortless Ways to Look 10 Years Younger, 10 Pounds Lighter, 10 Times Better by Charla Krupp (Springboard Press).

The Okinawa Program: Learn the Secrets to Healthy Longevity by Bradley Willcox, Craig Willcox and Makoto Suzuki (Three Rivers Press).

What's Age Got to Do with It?: Living Your Healthiest and Happiest Life by Robin McGraw (Thomas Nelson).

Younger Next Year for Women: Live Strong, Fit, and Sexy until You're 80 and Beyond by Chris Crowley and Henry S. Lodge, MD (Workman Publishing).

Aging is aging; inevitable, not always pleasant but ultimately something we must make peace with. The only way I see to do that is to start making amends with ourselves first. After that, aging is downright easy.

Princess Julia's
Pet Peeve #3: Rigidity

To be charming is to be flexible, impromptu, elastic, spontaneous; when you are rigid it closes you off to human emotion – yours, mine, the emotions of others. It's not something we talk a lot about these days, but you see rigidity everywhere: in the husband who won't hand over the remote, in the wife who won't watch football, in the kids who refuse to do their homework, in the friends who won't try your favorite Thai restaurant, in the family who won't support your lifestyle choice, in the neighbor who won't put out luminaries in the driveway (like everybody else) at the holidays. To be rigid is to miss golden opportunities that make life, and people, more CHARMing. So let go of the reins, take off your blinders, say yes to possibility, and experience for yourself what it means to truly embrace life on your own, CHARMing terms.

When Your Mid-life Crisis Lasts Longer Than Puberty

I read an article the other day called "Mid-Wife Crisis" about a woman so unhappy in her marriage she thought of divorce every single day. My first thought was, "Why is this woman still married?" Then I recalled how I felt when I first started to notice the initial signs of aging a couple years ago.

I couldn't imagine what was wrong with me. Was I sick? Had I been overdoing it? Why was I so sore, tired, cranky, irritable and puffy? Why did I suddenly have sinus problems and digestive issues and all sorts of other, unpleasant and spontaneous things going on with my body that weren't happening a year or two earlier?

It was less a mid-life crisis and more a mind-blowing experience: I wasn't a spring chicken anymore!

But in coming to terms with the calendar, I realized that no amount of whining, moaning, groaning, or plastic surgery was going to stop the inevitable onslaught of aging. So I faced up to it, owned it, embraced it and am a much better, much more CHARMing woman for it.

Parting Words About Aging

As we close the chapter on aging – literally and figuratively – I want to leave us feeling positive, hopeful and, above all, *youthful*. All I can say is this: when you age gracefully, you really do stay young at heart. This idea is not original with me, but I can't say it any better.

In the final analysis age is what we make of it. I've had my days where the mirror seems like a 3-D movie theater screen and picks up every laugh line, wrinkle, droop, and drag. Then, too, I've caught myself laughing, smiling, or joking in a passing reflection and am reminded of the school girl I was not so long ago. What's the difference? Just one thing: How I felt about what I saw.

And therein lies the secret remedy to aging. Don't spend so much time analyzing what you see, inspecting every line or crease, or obsessing over what used to be up here and is now down there. No matter how many procedures and potions you try you'll never be eighteen again. And, between you and me, who'd *want* to be?

I'd much rather be me, right now, today – who I am and where I've been and what I've seen and whom I've touched in this lifetime – than who I was back then. I'm much happier and actually feeling better about myself now than I ever did back then.

And that, my friends, is what aging can't take away from us: How we feel about who we are.

War on aging? Let me clue you in on a little secret: there is no war to be won except to live to a ripe old age in good health and good spirits. That is the only way to win the war with aging.

Remember, as long as you continue to age gracefully your sense of humor can't wrinkle, your good nature can't sag, your compassion can't dry up and your charm will never, ever tarnish because what's most beautiful about us is unequivocally timeless.

$$
\begin{array}{l}
\text{C} \\
\text{H}\ \text{allmarks are CHARMing} \\
\text{A} \\
\text{R} \\
\text{M}
\end{array}
$$

Hallmarks are CHARMing

"Always remember that you are absolutely unique. Just like everyone else."

Margaret Mead

While the word "hallmark" most likely brings to mind a greeting card these days, it's actually a term dating back to the 18th century when the Goldsmiths' Company of London, located in Goldsmiths' Hall, would mark silver and gold items with a special stamp to indicate their purity and verity. Since then, the term hallmark has come to mean any distinguishing characteristic or feature of a person, place, or thing, often a characteristic reflecting genuineness and high quality.

When we talk about the hallmark of a person, we are talking about what makes that person unique and recognizable – kind of a personal brand. Companies have brands, and logos that are a representation of those brands – Coke's striking red and white logo and global appeal of refreshment and fun, Apple's simple apple logo associated with innovation, cool gadgets and beautiful design, Nike's familiar swoosh symbol and connection with famous sports figures to remind that each consumer can take control of their own destiny. Why can't people have brands too?

Personal branding has become a big deal in the business world and in career management. As you will see in the next chapters, you don't have to be a high-powered executive or job seeker to benefit from a personal brand. Playing up your strengths, having a recognizable style, and always being true to who you are is having a personal brand. That is what I mean by Hallmarks, the personal mark of excellence which is a cornerstone of the CHARMing woman.

Chapter 4

Princess Julia on Style

"Fashions fade, style is eternal."

Yves Saint Laurent

Over the years I've tried to cultivate a signature style for myself. I recently asked a friend what she thinks of when she thinks of "Julia's style." She said that she can always count on me to have my hair done nicely, even on a casual day when it's stuck in a ponytail. She also notices that I wear pale colors, including a lot of pastels that go well with my blond hair and fair skin tone and light eyes, and that I dress in flowing, blousy tunic tops that look ultra-feminine and play up my cleavage. She also knows that I wear a lot of jewelry. Bingo! She spotted my style at once.

But did you notice that she talked only about my looks? What about my signature style from the inside out? Well, when I asked her about that, she said I am always cheerful and outgoing and that I always seem like I'm up for some fun but at the same time mean business, assuming there's business to get done. Bingo, again! She was right on the money with spotting my hallmarks.

Spotting Hallmarks

Now let's think about some people we all know – or at least think we know because they're so in the world spotlight. When I mention Angelina Jolie and Madonna, what comes to mind? What do they have in common, besides the fact that both are successful, affluent, mega stars in the entertainment world? You probably thought of their care and concern for disadvantaged or orphaned children, right? You may have thought of them as devoted mothers. But, what about the differences, especially in their styles?

Angelina is a stunning beauty who plays up her looks without really playing them up at all. She dresses in comfortable yet classic and elegant clothing. Her grooming is simple, with make-up and hairstyles that are natural and not fussy. Her style is consistent. All of those things are her hallmarks.

Then there's Madonna. Talk about a 180-degree difference in styles! While Madonna can do the classic, simple, elegant look, she might just as likely be found wearing fishnet stockings, combat boots, and her underwear on the outside of her clothes, including a bra made out of the pointiest cones. Her hallmark is that she is unpredictable – always reinventing herself with yet another creative look, pushing the boundary of good taste. By definition, a hallmark would usually be a consistent style, but Madonna is consistent in her inconsistency and therefore it has become one of her distinguishing characteristics. It's what we've come to expect of her. You with me?

The Kind of Hallmark You Don't
Put in an Envelope

So, let's look at what we now know about hallmarks. Our hallmarks are our "greeting card" to the world. They are the things that people know about us, from first impression to repeated encounters over time. And, like all aspects of CHARM, they derive from within and outside of us. They are our outer "look" – our style of dress and grooming, the manner in which we carry ourselves, our image on the surface. They are also an expression of our inner selves – a consistent way of being. They are an expression of who we truly are when we are at our best.

In this chapter, we'll focus on the outer hallmarks and my advice for living your life with style. Then, the next chapter will focus on your inner hallmarks.

It's Not Who You Wear,
But How You Wear It

Too many women get hung up on labels. If that suit doesn't have the right designer label on it, no matter how much the price tag is, they won't buy it. Sure, it's kinda neat to say "I'm wearing an Armani suit" and, most of the time, a really expensive suit will look, well, expensive, and the fine quality and cut will make you feel really good about yourself. But you know what? If you don't have CHARM, no matter what the price tag was for that suit, or whose name is sewn into the jacket, it won't matter if you can't pull it off.

That's because style is an attitude, not a thing; it's how you act, not what you wear. I can look around a room full of impeccably dressed, coiffed and manicured women and spot those with true style. And usually they're not wearing the most expensive outfit or dripping in the priciest jewelry.

Style is what happens when you're wearing your clothes, when you're washing your clothes, when you're buying your clothes – and when you're buck naked. You can put CHARMing women in a potato sack and they'd still have style.

Style starts with confidence, builds with knowledge, grows with practice, and eventually blossoms into how you walk, talk, think, act, and just plain are. But unlike the fashion of the moment, there is a timeless elegance in the individually expressed actions and tastes of the CHARMing woman, and that is what I mean by Style.

Style Isn't Something You "Get," It's Something You "Have"

Many women think they can happen upon style, buy style, beg, or borrow it, but already they're going about it the wrong way because style begins from within. It's personal and powerful because you literally "own" it. In short, style isn't something you "get," it's something you "have."

I'm not saying style can't be learned; it can. But for style to stick it must be felt, deep inside, where it really counts. You can attend all the fashion shows and galas in the world, watch *What Not to Wear* and *Project Runway* until your eyes cross, but if you're not passionate about learning what style is and isn't – in cultivating your own individual expression of taste – it simply won't stick and you'll be right back where you started.

More than what you wear, style is how you wear something; it's not what you do but how you do it. Style is an offshoot of our personality, a way of acting, thinking, and unconsciously being, even when we're not actively thinking about it. How do you describe cool? You don't; it just is. Same goes with style.

You can call Tina Turner a diva, but what does that really mean? You can call Grace Kelly elegant, but how do you define that? How do you pinpoint what makes Tina a diva or Grace an icon? How do you break it down? Is it the hair, the eyes, hats, makeup, heels, or hips? It is all of those things, some of those things, and none of those things. It is how those women put them together in a consistent manner. That's style, plain and simple.

I could dress like Tina Turner or Grace Kelly and it would always just look like a Halloween costume. Not because I'm unattractive or unworthy, but because their styles simply aren't

Princess Julia's
CHARM Tip #4

Pick one thing and make it your signature. Maybe you almost always wear a great jacket or scarf, or always have a distinctive hairstyle that you wear consistently, or come to be known for wearing unique artisan jewelry.

my style. Style is ultimately personal and absolutely unique to you. Sure, say the names Bette Davis, Katherine Hepburn, and Lauren Bacall and you get the same basic type of style – classic, ladylike, sophisticated – but each woman had her own unique way of being classic, ladylike, and sophisticated. Bette Davis was cool and aloof, Hepburn was part debutante and part tomboy, while Bacall is seventeen types of sultry. So, what's your style?

A *Style Questionnaire*

To help you pinpoint your own personal style, fill in the blanks beside each question below. This is far from scientific and while I'm no Tim Gunn, I think by the time you've filled out a half dozen or so blanks you'll start to get a feel for your own personal style:

- The color that appeals to me most is…
- I'm happiest when I wear…
- Being comfortable is more important than…
- If I had unlimited money I would wear…
- If I were at my perfect weight or fitness level, I would wear…
- My favorite heel height is…
- When it comes to hair, I like…
- I'd rather wear sunglasses than…
- I am most comfortable in…
- Sweatpants are for…

- My favorite style icon is…
- I also really admire…
- My favorite outfit I wear now is…
- My favorite outfit I've ever owned is…
- If I could wear anything at all formal it would be…
- If I could wear anything at all informal it would be…

Putting Your Style Into Practice

What good is it to know your style if you don't work it? Now that you have a better sense of what type of accessories, attitude, and apparel are right for you, it's time to start folding them into your everyday life.

Start by investing in accessories and apparel that are more appropriate for who you really are. Don't break the bank right away; take your time. In fact, the slower you take this process the more natural it will feel for you and look for everybody else.

Next, take pains to get comfortable in your own skin. If a new hair color is part of your new style, own it, work it, love it, and live it. If high heels are something you're not used to, but are really enjoying, I can tell you that the more you wear them, the easier they get to walk in.

Finally, be proud – openly proud – of your new sense of style. The more comfortable you get with it, the more proud you'll be. Remember that even if you don't get a total makeover or buy one new stitch of clothing, you can still embrace your own personal style – and be charming doing it!

Princess Julia's Favorite Books on Style

Freakin' Fabulous: How to Dress, Speak, Behave, Eat, Drink, Entertain, Decorate, and Generally Be Better than Everyone Else by Clinton Kelly (Simon Spotlight Entertainment).

How to Have Style by Isaac Mizrahi (Gotham).

The Little Black Book of Style by Nina Garcia (Collins Living).

The One Hundred: A Guide to the Pieces Every Stylish Woman Must Own by Nina Garcia (Collins Living).

Tim Gunn: A Guide to Quality, Taste, and Style by Tim Gunn and Kate Maloney (Abrams Image).

Princess Julia's Quick Tips on Style

Now that I've got you hungry for style, here are some more, general "quick tips" to make you more stylish – and charming – than ever:

1. If you have charm, a well-tailored suit will make you look as presidential as any corporate woman or politician. Remember that clothes don't make the woman, the woman makes the clothes.

2. If you must have a designer label, either go to a high-end resale shop, a discount store, or web site that carries designer

labels – or at least buy it on sale! You don't need to pay full price! Style is as much about planning as it is about purchasing.

3. Buy outfits that are timeless and are staples in your closet – a good suit that crosses over from work to going out at night, the essential little black dress, well-tailored slacks that can be worn for a few seasons with new tops, etc. Make sure that all new purchases reflect your own personal style.

4. Don't buy trendy clothes – and don't buy clothes too young, or too old, for you. Dress your age. Don't follow fashion; create your own!

5. Invest in good shoes, earrings, a purse, and watch that can be used or worn for years and years and years. Let your CHARM rub off on these and you will carry that CHARM for years to come.

The Three Elements of Style

Style comes in many shapes and sizes, but after decades in the beauty industry, I have boiled style down to three basic elements that any woman can have and enjoy. They are:

✳ Confidence

It's listed first because just as concrete makes for the solid foundation of a house, confidence is the first ingredient for knockout style. In fact, I dare you to show me someone who is stylish *and* unconfident. It simply can't happen. Even nebbish notables like Woody Allen and Bob Newhart have a particular style; that's because they're so confident in what they do well that it rubs off in how they look, what they wear, and even how they act. Confidence lets you roam freely throughout your own style, buying what you like versus what everybody else is buying and helping you pull off whatever you put on with style. Confidence makes you stylish even when your size or shape put you at odds with the norm. Look at Queen Latifah, self-described as "big, black, and beautiful" and pulling it all off with style to spare, not to mention other trendsetters like *Ugly Betty's* America Ferrara and *Dancing With the Star's* Cheryl Burke.

✳ Character

You can't possibly know your own personal style if you don't know who you are, if you aren't familiar with, let alone comfortable with, your own content and character. Knowing who you are, in fact, is the first step to finding and living your own personal style. Character is what lies at the very heart of you; it's what you do and how you act and where you go and who you are when nobody is watching. It's your default setting, your base level, and your status quo. Whether it's a quiet, contemplative thinker, a free spirit, a philosopher, a poet, or a princess, your character is what lies at the heart of you – and what dictates your every move. To know your personal character is to build upon the solid foundation of moral and ethical strength.

✳ Class

Lastly, class rounds out the three elements of style. That's because no matter how you dress, you can still have class. No matter where you live, what you do, how much you weigh or what you believe in, you can hold your head high, act with confidence, live with character, and walk with class. Class is the calm in the storm, the knowing smile in the face of setback. It's the turning of the other cheek when others strike back. It's taking the high road when others veer into the gutter, and a mannerly response to rudeness. Like style, like CHARM, class is something that exists at your core where it rightfully belongs.

Princess Julia's
Pet Peeve #4: Not Dressing Your Age

No matter what your signature style is, make sure it's age-appropriate. A style can be classic and elegant, casual and funky, wacky and creative, or anything you want it to be. Just don't dress younger than you are. Nothing wrong with having a touch of youth in your look – you don't need to go frumpy and matronly at any age, no matter how advanced in years. But, overall keep your style relevant and flattering for your age.

Parting Words About Style

CHARM is what polishes you off. You can be wearing an expensive outfit from head to toe, but if you don't have charm, you won't pull it off and it just won't feel right. That's because CHARM is all about feelings; just like style.

We always focus on the clothes, hair, makeup, and accessories, but those are only the icing on the cake. Style is not so much what we wear but how we wear it. Style begins with intuition and develops through acquisition, but the key to a personal sense of style is to accent the personal; style begins and ends with your individual imprint.

Style is "confidence in clothes." It's you being you, no matter what fashion says, people think, or even say. Even if your style is to ignore fashion (for now) and focus on things that are more important to you, guess what? That's still your style – your hallmark -- and we love you for it!

Chapter 5

Princess Julia on Honesty and Being Yourself

"*If you tell the truth you don't have to remember anything.*"

Mark Twain

When I started my business and formulated my skincare products, I knew I wanted to base my enterprise on honesty and total respect for the consumer. With all my experience in the cosmetics industry, I knew that it was possible to formulate a good quality product that I could sell at a reasonable price. I invested as much as possible in research and development, in sourcing the best possible ingredients, and developed a packaging that protects the product but doesn't break the bank. I wanted to be able to sleep with a clear conscience at night. I'm here to tell you, I do!

I don't think it's possible to be a CHARMing person without honesty and the best place to start is by being honest with yourself! We women tend to nit pick at our own imperfections. We tell ourselves we're not as qualified as we really are, not as pretty, not as smart, not as worthy, not as funny, wise, or fun to be around. The more lies you tell yourself, the easier it is to tell lies to others – and the harder it is to be CHARMing.

If we keep doing that, we won't ever be honest with or about ourselves, with anyone or about anything! And if you can't be honest, your CHARM level will sink to new lows. That's because CHARM is about authenticity -- the true and honest emotions you feel day in, day out.

Now, the thing about honesty is that we don't have very many good role models when it comes to telling the truth. Celebrities get caught lying all the time, so do reporters, CEOs, businesspeople, politicians, and even presidents. So it's easy to get caught up in the trend of dishonesty, fudging on your taxes, or making up excuses for why you can't get to work on time, or where you've been when your husband asks.

But the path from honesty to dishonesty is a slippery slope. I have several colleagues who couldn't be nicer people, and yet I find them fibbing more and more often about completely irrelevant things: what movie they saw, who they went out to dinner with, how much money they make. Are these really things we want to lose our integrity over?

We all think "white lies" are little things, and they are – at first. But white lies grow like snowballs. The more you tell, the

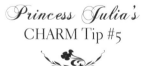

Princess Julia's
CHARM Tip #5

When you're contemplating telling a "harmless" little white lie versus telling the truth, imagine what you say being broadcast on the evening news or posted all over the Internet. Wouldn't you rather be known for honesty?

bigger – and easier – they are to tell. A fib here, a fib there, and pretty soon we're telling more lies than truth. And how charming is that?

A Half Truth is a Whole Lie

The problem with honesty is that we all think we can play fast and loose with it. Some of that is societal. I mean, do we really need to point out that girlfriend's gained some weight? Do we really need to tell hubby those too-short swim trunks make him look a tad chunky? And if we were to tell our kids what we really thought of what they wear to school every day, well, it could take years to undo those emotional scars. But there is a difference between omitting how we feel about something and actively telling someone something other than the truth.

For instance, let's say a coworker you can't stand asks you out for drinks after work. As always, there are two ways to handle this – with honesty and without. Without honesty, you might immediately come up with some lame excuse like, "Oh, sorry Sylvia, I've got to go watch my son's basketball game tonight." Now, maybe you have a son, maybe you don't. Maybe he plays basketball, maybe he's on the chess club. Whatever; it's not the details of the lie that matter but the lie itself. A second, more truthful option might be to say something like, "You know what, Sylvia, that sounds nice but I've been working so many overtime hours lately I'd just rather go home and spend time with my family. Can I take a rain check?"

Now both excuses are, well, excuses, but the first is an out-and-out fabrication and the second is the truth. Which one feels better to tell? And on the CHARM side, which is more thoughtful and kind to Sylvia? Which excuse do you think she'd rather hear?

Realistically speaking, if you're not honest about where Sylvia ranks on your priority list, she's likely to think that she still has a shot at happy hour. I mean, if you don't communicate honestly with her about how you prefer to spend your time, how will she ever come to realize that you'd rather do just about anything than go out with her? And that's absolutely your choice.

Part of being CHARMing is being honest with your emotions, your family, your friends, and about how you spend your time. Yes, of course, we all have to do things we don't want in this world – and that's no reason to be anything less than CHARMing when we do. However, if you're the kind of person who can't say "no" and always ends up doing things she doesn't really want to do, tension is going to build, your blood pressure is going to rise and your CHARMing quotient is going to go down accordingly.

Being sensitive but honest frees you up to live your own life on your terms. When you back yourself into corners with little white lies, questionable excuses, and out-and-out untruths, you do both yourself and the person you're being dishonest with a great disservice.

The Honesty Quiz

Below are a few simple statements, the kinds we make as modern human beings every day of the week. Some of them are untrue; others are honest expressions. Next to each statement you'll find a "D" for dishonest or an "H" for honest; circle the corresponding letter to decided whether the state is dishonest ("D) or honest ("H").

There's no grade, no fierce examination of each statement or judgment about which was which. By the end of the quiz, I think you'll find it easy to see which statements were honest and which were dishonest. Next, ask yourself, "Which statement is more CHARMing?" My guess is you'll know the answer right away.

So here goes:

• "I'd love to go to that play with you, Susie, but my husband's going to surprise me with a romantic dinner that night."	D	H
• "Can we do it next week, Sally? I'm just feeling really rundown and wouldn't be very good company."	D	H
• "Didn't I tell you I was going back to school, Ed? I've got classes every night of the week, and weekends too, for just about forever!"	D	H
• "I've got to be out of town on business that night, Ed, and for the foreseeable future. Sorry."	D	H
• "I wish I hadn't just put my grandmother in the nursing home last week, John. It's just going to be a really bad few months for us..."	D	H

• "Sally, manning the dunking booth at the county fair would be a real honor, but I've got jury duty that day. Yes, I know, for weekend court; it's something new..."	D	H
• "Let's do it next week, Brian. I've got a ton of errands to run and I know that's a lame excuse, but the fridge is empty and I've got lots of laundry to do if I'm going to have anything to wear to work tomorrow."	D	H
• "I'd love to, Bob, but I'm just swamped at work. Can I take a raincheck?	D	H

Princess Julia's Quick Tips on Honesty

Honesty begins with us; how we view the world – and particularly ourselves. It colors how we look at, talk to, and treat other people. So if we can't be honest with ourselves – about our strengths, our weaknesses, our vulnerabilities, our passions – how can we ever hope to be honest with others?

What's the big deal about honesty? Why is it so important? In a word, honesty is the glue that holds community together. It's what builds trust in a relationship and creates authentic conversations that actually mean something. Too often we translate the glib, sarcastic, backstabbing banality of TV conversations into our own lives, where they definitely don't belong.

Real life is for real people, and in the real world, real people communicate truthfully, honestly, and passionately with

Princess Julia's (Favorite Books on Honesty, Ethics, Marketing Yourself

Ethics For the New Millenium by the Dalai Lama (Riverhead Press).

Managing Brand You: 7 Steps to Creating Your Most Successful Self by Jerry S. Wilson and Ira Blumenthal (AMACOM).

Seven Days to Online Networking (Chapter 2: How to Stand Out in the Cyberspace Crowd) by Ellen Sautter and Diane Crompton (JIST).

Honest Business: Superior Strategy for Starting & Managing Your Own Business by Michael Phillips and Salli Rapberry (Clear Glass Publications)

each other. When honesty becomes optional, communication suffers, and so does character.

Not to worry. The quick tips below will help you become more honest with yourself and, in the process, more honest with others.

✳ Embrace Your Imperfections!

Look at yourself, inside and out, and recognize that you are not perfect–but you're working on it. And then realize that others are working on themselves in the exact same way. Remember that the lies we tell ourselves become the foundation for the lies we tell others, and when everyone is lying who is left to know the real truth?

❈ Don't Let Anger Control You

Instead, use anger to get over a situation, work through your feelings, and let CHARM ooze out through every pore. And remember to breathe the whole time, too! Control is the source from which honesty springs. Often, we get backed into fibbing by someone putting us on the spot or asking us to commit at that very moment. What do we do? We typically panic and will say anything to get out of it. When you are in control of your emotions – including anger – you are less likely to be put on the spot because you can now think on your feet. As a result, you are more likely to tell the truth without hurting someone else's feelings or your own credibility.

❈ Experience Your Feelings

Don't push them back in your mind. Feelings are natural; how you feel is never wrong, only how you react to those feelings by shoving them down in your stomach or burying them with alcohol, shopping, or food. The more we experience our feelings and allow them to see the light of day, the easier they are to cope with and the more honest we'll be with ourselves – and others.

❈ Encourage Yourself to Do What You Want to Do in Your Life!

And enjoy it! When we are firing on all cylinders, living the life we've always dreamed of, and working passionately with people we care about, it is easy to be honest about how we really

Princess Julia's
Pet Peeve #5: Fear

Fear kills CHARM sure as anger kills kindness. Now, there is a difference between being afraid of a legitimate fear, being fearful of the daily little things that can ruin a happy, productive life, and those that exist only in your mind, such as anticipations or what ifs.

Fear halts your progress, stops you in your tracks and forces you to re-examine everything you know and love. Confront your fears-- check against reality-- you can't be CHARMing, let alone yourself, when you're constantly worried about who's talking about you behind your back, what's happening with your job, or if your tire might get a flat while you're in the movie theater. We have plenty of real things to worry about. Stop "borrowing trouble," as my mother used to say, and don't worry about those things that aren't worthy of your stress, anxiety, and outright fear. Save your energy for the real issues that require your attention for final resolution. Work on complex issues by dividing them into small tasks that you can clear off one at a time.

feel. It is only when we live in denial – about our jobs, our hopes, our dreams – that we live a life of dishonesty and despair. You don't have to be in Hollywood or be a rock star to begin living your dreams. You can start right now, today, by being more open and honest about how you want to live your life and then taking active steps to live that way. What are you waiting for, anyway?

❋ Revisit Your Dreams

What did you want to do when you were younger? Are you doing, or have you done, what you dreamed about? If not, be honest about whether you're happy with what you are doing or have done. It's important to face up to where we are in life and where we want to be. Honesty is often the first thing to go when we're unhappy or unfulfilled, so it only stands to reason that the more fulfilled we are, the happier – and more honest – we'll be.

Parting Words about Honesty

At the very core of CHARM is honesty because you simply can't be fully CHARMing if you aren't fully honest. You will always be holding back, always be fudging just a little, if you don't look yourself in the mirror and lay it all on the line, honestly and truthfully.

What is it about you that causes you to fib, fudge, or just plain lie? Is it your job, your marriage, your body, your looks, your finances or your role in life? Pinpoint what it is that you are dishonest about most and take that out and analyze it until you can really face that demon honestly.

If it's your job, be honest about your career choice and look for alternatives that will make you happy. If it's your body, join a gym or get a personal trainer to begin exploring how to be honest in that area of your life. If it's money, consider how much you spend and get that area of your life under control so you can approach it more honestly.

Whatever it is you're being dishonest about will continue to haunt you if you don't face up to it and tackle it head on. That is what honesty is all about; stripping away the trappings and getting down to the nitty-gritty.

Once you can be honest with yourself, you'll find it almost impossible to express dishonesty to others. And, finally, you can begin walking the path back to CHARMing again. If you've lost your CHARM, look to honesty first. That's where you're likely to find it hiding, and that's where you'll find your true hallmarks.

C
H
Altruism is CHARMing
R
M

Altruism is CHARMing

"Helping people in need is a good and essential part of my life, a kind of destiny."
Diana Princess of Wales

The chapters in this section might be my favorite in the whole book! You see, altruism – doing good for others, being generous, charitable, and caring – is what makes my version of CHARM different from the old-fashioned notion of "charm." The old version of charm could be quite selfish. It was about using your wiles, your looks, and superficial aspects of your personality to win over others so that you could get something from them. There was a time during the reign of my grandparents when charm was a weapon to be used in getting people to do your bidding or a trick to gain entrance into upper levels of society.

My CHARM, on the other hand, is about being as beautiful on the inside as the outside so that I can make other people feel the same way. So, altruism may represent just one letter of the five letters in the acronym "CHARM," but it's a truly important one! Without altruism, there is no CHARM.

Chapter 6

Princess Julia on Community and Caring

> "In a democratic society we must live cooperatively, and serve the community in which we live, to the best of our ability. For our own success to be real, it must contribute to the success of others."
>
> Eleanor Roosevelt

Imagine being European royalty, living in a mansion surrounded by luxury – furs, evening gowns, jewels, servants at your beck and call, all the stereotypical regal stuff. One day that's your life; the next day you're on a crowded, stinking ship with barely enough food to eat, making the rough passage to America. You go from being members of Hungary's former ruling family – a prince and princess – to being a coal miner and housewife in West Virginia.

Sound like the kind of fiction that would make a great Disney or Steven Spielberg film? Maybe so, but it's fact, not fiction. That was the life of my Karoly grandparents who fled Hungary with all their possessions in two suitcases to escape certain assassination when the Karoly family's rule was overthrown by Communists in the 1919 revolution.

Soon after landing in New York, my grandparents moved to West Virginia, where a strong Hungarian population had cropped up. There, they adjusted to a hard, but happy, life. When I was a child, my grandmother would often tell me how she learned the importance of community and how family, neighbors, good friends, and other loved ones are the most important things in life – not the jewelry, receptions, and breakfast in bed on silver trays.

In your efforts to become more CHARMing, your work won't be complete until you factor service to your community into your life, if you haven't already. I don't mean just writing a check to a charity or stopping by a soup kitchen to dish up lunches for a few minutes. Those things count – every little bit counts, in fact – and I'm not here to judge what is or isn't worthwhile to society. But, what I do mean by community service is caring for others on a regular basis – caring for others the way the Hungarians in exile in West Virginia cared for my grandparents during their time of need. The community cared enough to teach them the basic skills they needed in this new life. But it was thanks to my grandparents' extraordinary upbringing and education that they were able to give back to their community and make important contributions at every level. You see, community service is about care and respect – making people feel loved, supported and valued.

Community is Everywhere

Community is made up of every person you come into contact with – friends, family, co-workers, customers, sales people, neighbors, teachers, and the list goes on and on. So, while you might think of doing community service as going out to an area of your town or city to work with people who need your help, usually under the auspices of a formal charitable organization, community service is really about helping and caring for anyone who needs you.

At some point in your life, you might spend a great deal of time caring for an aging or sick loved one and not have any time left over to do traditional volunteer work. That's more than okay, it's wonderful. At other times, you might find that your opportunities to help the people close to you – friends, family, neighbors – are limited. Everyone's doing okay and fending for themselves! Those are the times when you ought to look for formal volunteer opportunities beyond your own backyard.

Those Cavemen Were CHARMing!

Ages ago all we had was each other. We roamed the earth in tribes, hunting and gathering in those close-knit groups. Often it took a whole village to take down a huge beast, skin it, clean it, cook the meat, and sew the skins into clothes for one and all. When there was food, we all ate; when there was no food, we starved together.

Later, caves gave way to walls and rooms separated by fences and hedges, and hunting and gathering turned into classes and divisions. Then came the rich and the poor, the city and the farm, downtowns and suburbs, subdivisions and mansions. Communities grew larger but the sense of community grew smaller and smaller until, these days, you're lucky if you know one or two neighbors.

With that breakdown in community came a real loss. Now we know TV stars better than we know people on our own street, in the grocery stores, or at church. One can sit back and trace the breakdown of CHARM along with the destruction of our city, state, and local communities.

That can change, but only if you make it happen. Unfortunately, what most of us do is take steps to close ourselves off more and more from our community, not leaving ourselves open to new relationships, experiences, and neighbors. Think of how we treat each other – the crass and sarcastic words we use with family, friends, and loved ones, the impatience we show to the checkout girl or bag boy, the fingers we snap to get the waiter's attention and how we revel in sending a message about his or her poor service through a smaller tip. Is this CHARMing? Hardly.

Burning Bridges Leaves You with No Way Back to CHARM

The problem with treating others disrespectfully – besides that it is just plain morally wrong – is that the disrespect is only going to come back to hit us in the face. No woman is an island unto herself. We can't exist without community – no matter how big or small that may be. We need each other, and not just for hurricane relief or for someone to bring us our chicken cordon bleu at a fancy restaurant.

Like it or not, we are all linked to each other by how we act, what we do, and even what we say. True charm is the great equalizer; you treat everyone the same, from busboy to billionaire, from supermarket checkout clerk to supermodel, from family member to stranger.

I know it's easy to be short, be impatient, get frustrated, to snap. Heaven knows, in this day and age, too many of us are on short fuses. But when you feel free to let loose on underlings or those you consider "outside your circle," you are merely debasing yourself by showing your lack of class, grace, and charm. We must all be good to each other. When you fuss, fight, and burn bridges in your community, you leave yourself no route back to CHARM, and that's a very lonely place indeed.

Princess Julia's
CHARM Tip #6

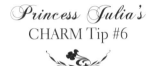

Never let a single day go by without committing at least one act of kindness, whether it's a day of volunteer work or a five-minute phone call to check on a friend who's been feeling down, or a lonely relative.

Circles of Care, Ripples of Relief

Like most things to be CHARMing about, community starts with you. Don't wait until the ripples in the pond of community reach you; cause those ripples yourself. Be the force of change in your community – no matter how large or small.

You can lead by example, and it doesn't take much. Start with a smile. It's free, it's good exercise (yes, it really is!), and it's downright contagious. Once a day I try an experiment with someone new – a growling teenager, a frowning waiter, a scowling gas station attendant, or a grumpy friend. I see their anger, fear, resentment, or disappointment from a mile off as they approach and ready myself with a strong look in the eye, a cheerful outlook, and a big, wide smile. It's not scientific, but trust me, nine out of ten times you'll get a smile in return. And in a lot of cases, it's just what's needed to turn a day around.

If a smile doesn't work, or isn't enough, say something nice.

Frenzied wait staff stop and listen if you let them know they're doing a good job, and who doesn't like it when you notice their new haircut, that last few pounds they lost, or that they bought a new purse?

If talking doesn't help, lend an ear. Listening is one of the greatest ways to embrace your community. People sometimes just want to talk. Doesn't matter who we are, what we do or where we're from, we're all the same. We just want someone to listen. If you can take two or three minutes out of your day to ask a friend, a colleague, a server, a cashier, a hairdresser how their day is going, you can further embrace your community one problem at a time.

So you see, it's not difficult to change yourself, your community, or even the world with just a few simple measures – a smile, a kind word, or a warm touch.

Remember, it's not the big things that equal CHARM but the small, everyday steps you take to make your world a better place, one smile, conversation, or embrace at a time.

Princess Julia's
Favorite Books on Community and Caring

Deliberate Acts of Kindness: Service as a Spiritual Practice by Meredith Gould (Image).

Volunteer Vacations: Short Term Adventuress That Will Benefit You and Others by Bill McMillon, Doug Cutchins, Anne Geissinger (Chicago Review Press).

How Can I Help? Stories and Reflection on Service by Ram Dass and Paul Gorman (Knopf).

The Joy of Volunteering: Working and Surviving in Developing Countries by Othniel J. Seiden (Books to Believe In).

Creating With Others: The Practice of Imagination in Life, Art, and the Workplace by Shaun McNiff

And imagine what a difference you can make if you add formal volunteer work in your community-at-large!

Princess Julia's Quick Tips on Community

As we wind down our chapter on the importance of caring for your community, here are a few of my quick tips to remind you how easy it is to improve your own little corner of the world:

❋ Remember the Six Degrees of Separation Rule

"I'm rubber, you're glue. Whatever you say bounces off me and sticks to you." This childhood saying is relevant to our conversation about community because what you say and do really does circle back to you. Much as you can change a person's day with a smile or a kind word, you can also ruin it with a frown or a put-down. The ways in which negativity and pettiness ripple through a community and circle back are countless – and none of them is good. Remember that we are all connected, and that you are only six people away from contacting any other person on this shrinking planet. So be cautious as you make your way through life: every word, thought and action sets off a chain of reactions, all of which comes back home to you.

❋ Learn to Accept People for Who They Are

We all have different roles to play and jobs to do while on this planet, and who's to say which are important or not. You never know if your waiter is working his way through Harvard or if the local community organizer is going to be the next president. Whatever a person is or isn't shouldn't affect how you treat them. CHARM treats everyone the same way – and that way is open, honest and caring.

❋ Be CHARMing at All Times

No matter what others may say or do, you control how CHARMing you are, and your treatment of others should not depend on a person's religion, race, or social standing. That is why CHARM is so much more than a nice suit or good manners.

I've seen women cut people down with a smile on their face and a seam in their slacks, but there's nothing CHARMing about the words coming out of their mouths or the evil eye they're giving. CHARM comes from within, and you are in control of how you treat people at all times. Never forget that CHARM can change lives; it truly can – beginning with yours and those in your community.

❊ Don't Judge

You can disagree with something someone says or does without being judgmental. Your CHARM will allow them to see you as nice and non-aggressive, not a threat to them. "Agreeing to disagree" is the sign of a true adult and someone so interested in fostering relationships within her community that she is willing to overlook a personal point of view, while respecting her feelings, to understand and relate to the other person.

❊ Relationships are Built in Communities

Relationships aren't like construction sites where you never know whether you'll fall in a hole or find a detour. They're more like paved interstates that go for the long haul. Sure, you might need to rest and refuel now and again, but the fact that it's a relationship implies that you'll be back on the journey before too long. CHARM is the long haul. Anyone can be funny or trite or "on" for a few minutes, a few hours, or even a few days, but a few days does not a relationship make. By being consistently CHARMing you fully commit to the relationship, and the others can't help but commit as well.

If you don't like me, fine; that's one thing. But if you can't tolerate me, well, we're going to have issues. Intolerance, to my way of thinking, is just another form of arrogance; you're too good for me, don't have enough time for me or, what's worse, don't have any interest whatsoever in what I'm saying.

People who are intolerant are no better than people who are angry; there is something going on inside them that destroys any chance they have at being CHARMing. For them, CHARM is a plastered-on smile, strong, firm, clammy handshake and pretending to be listening as they wait for our mouths to stop moving so they can hurry up and say something more important. We know better, and that's why to be CHARMing is to be tolerant of everyone.

Parting Words about Community

CHARM will allow you to accept everyone for who they are as they enter and leave your daily routine – or life! The best part about CHARM and community is that you won't judge them based on a word said, an action taken or the way they dress.

If you still have lingering doubts about the power of CHARM in your community, just ask yourself this simple question: "What if everyone read this book and acted more CHARMing?" Could you imagine a life more CHARMing? A life where everyone is treated with respect? Where everyone complimented each other authentically and realistically? Where everyone was patient, understanding, and concerned? Where everyone made time to care for the neighbor in need, whether that neighbor is the elderly woman next door they've known for years or a stranger in a homeless shelter?

Such is the potential for a community based on CHARM rather than crass, greedy, or selfish behavior. Sure, we're a long way from that at the moment, but it only takes a few CHARMing people to get the ball rolling and the rest may join in. Won't you be one of those CHARMers right now?

Chapter 7

Princess Julia on
Wealth and Abundance

"The safe way to double your money is to fold it over once and put it in your pocket."

Frank Hubbard

My grandmother Karoly – the same one I told you about in Chapter 6, the one who went from riches to rags when she and my grandfather immigrated to the United States – loved to teach me life lessons when I was little. One thing she often talked about was the importance of money, or why money actually isn't all that important. She'd gone from having a royal treasury to wracking poverty and she claimed she was happier when she didn't have as much. Not having any at all was very difficult, and she taught me the value of the middle ground, the wisdom of knowing when enough is enough.

My grandma was pregnant with my Uncle John while she was on that miserable ocean voyage to the new world, and she gave birth shortly after arriving in America. She had more children while living the difficult life of a coal miner's wife in West Virginia. So her new life in the new world was all about family – not something she'd had much of when she lived in the lap of luxury in Budapest. While in the old country they had all sorts of tutors and nannies, but now she was the one responsible for instilling her solid values in her young children, making sure they were disciplined and had a proper upbringing and education.

To my grandmother, family was everything. As long as she had a happy, healthy family close to her, she felt blessed with abundance. So, my first lessons about wealth were that "it's not about the money."

Let Me Make Something Abundantly Clear

When people hear the word "abundance" they immediately think money. And when they think money, they think *a lot* of money! The working and middle classes think that because they don't have Donald Trump's money, they're not rich, or that they don't have abundance in their life. But abundance isn't just money; it's much more valuable than that.

Abundance is having a rich life filled with love and joy, caring friends and loving family, pets that love you and children who adore you, a fulfilling job – even if it's not a highly-paid position – and hobbies like gardening or exhilarating sports that let you experience life in all its glory and on your own terms. It all boils down to determining your life priorities and placing your efforts behind achieving them. Money itself is just the result of work. But love, happiness, wisdom, companionship, you name them– can you buy those? And abundance comes by attracting those "riches" to you – in the most CHARMing way possible, of course. And just what do you do with that abundance you bring to yourself? You do the altruistic thing – you share it!

The "Real" Power of Attraction

Most of the people I know with lots and lots of money have very little CHARM. And how could they? They're too busy making money. There's no gardening for them, no quality time with the family, no romantic getaways or *Sex & the City* marathons on DVD, or lost weekends, or time enough to sit and reflect on life, love, and happiness.

Abundance does not mean Money. Abundance is gaving enough of what you need. Look up the word in the dictionary and you will not find the mention of money in the definition of Abundance. Neither is money the real power of attraction. The real power of attraction is CHARM; sending out positive, loving, caring, trusting, listening, empowering, altruistic vibes that radiate through others and come back to you in ways as yet untold or even imagined.

You are the one who controls how abundant and satisfying your life is. Through your actions – through your CHARM – you dictate life's terms; you don't sit and wait for it to be doled out to you. When I get up in the morning I don't wonder if I'll have a good day; I'm certain of it because I create my surroundings, I establish my priorities, and I generate energy and enthusiasm in the way I treat myself, my job, my company, my family, my friends, and my world.

You know by now that CHARM is not just a folded napkin, or a thank you note, or a glittering party invitation. CHARM is a core default setting that looks out at life with style, grace, calm, and confidence. It is a way of life, not just a happy accident or occasional fluke. CHARMing is as CHARMing does, and in a revolving door of gratitude and openness the more CHARM you give, the more CHARM you get back. Yes, it really *is* just that simple.

Five Tips for Inviting Abundance

When you invite abundance into your life, charm will allow you to become a conduit of grace, attracting abundance in every part of your life. This abundance may come in the form of a job promotion, new friend, fascinating conversation, heartwarming experience, spontaneous life lesson, or sometimes just a quiet, thoughtful moment of appreciation and serenity.

Abundance can come when you least expect it or as the result of careful planning. Remember that abundance isn't just money, fame, or possessions but the richness of life experiences that come from radiating charm 24-7-365. And, yes, it might even come in the form of money! You can use CHARM to invite abundance by:

✳ Investing Time

Invest time in relationships, jobs, hobbies – and yourself – to increase abundance. This investment may not pay off immediately, but you'll know it when the number of your friendships increases, your work prospers and the ties that bind your family become stronger.

Time is your most valuable resource. You can always get your money back, but you can't get your time back. Invest it wisely. Identify time wasters–internet surfing, television–and swap them out for more productive endeavors.

❋ Accepting and Loving Yourself First

Allow yourself to open up and invite abundance into your life. Abundance, like CHARM itself, starts within. You can't receive if you can't give, and you can't give if you don't feel worthy to share your gifts with the world at large. Self-acceptance is the surest way to find true abundance.

❋ Recognizing that CHARM Gets You Through Suffering

Even during the low times, CHARM will allow you to survive and still have a life full of riches and abundance. We all suffer through the highs and lows of life. The ups and downs aren't just part of living but are life lessons, one and all. It all depends on how you deal with the situation, maintaining a constructive attitude of searching for a solution, of seeking help when you can't figure out how to resolve an issue. By understanding that you can make the best of a bad situation, your life can be abundant even when your bank account isn't!

❋ Believing that Money Doesn't Buy Happiness

You've heard that all your life, but do you really believe it? On some level, we all know money can't buy happiness – or love! – but don't we all harbor some secret belief that we *would* be happier if only we had more money? This is true for people who are already swimming in dough as well as those living hand to mouth.

I know it's a hard concept to swallow, but sometimes less is actually more – more contentment, that is. We have been so trained by the media, entertainment, and other influences around us to equate money with abundance, but the two are like apples and oranges. Both taste sweet but are fundamentally different. Believe that happiness and money can be independent of each other and you immediately become richer in the bargain.

✳ Understanding Giving and Accepting

Accept what is offered to you with dignity. It can be hard for us to accept the blessings we've been given. How hard is it for us to accept a compliment, let someone buy us lunch, or treat us to a girl's night out? Sometimes the only way to appreciate giving is to receive in return, and when you can be okay with that – when receiving is as easy as giving –abundance can enter your life and stay there for good.

Investing in Yourself Pays Huge Dividends

As the financial planners say, we often pay ourselves last. That means we're so busy stressing about our job and socking away for our futures that we forget to treat ourselves now and again.

We've already heard how investing in yourself can pay off in abundance, but what does that really mean? Think of your life as the ultimate career, bank account, IRA, or stock. It is *that* valuable. You can have all the money in the world but if you don't have your health, happiness, family, freedom, and friends what do you really have at all?

My friend runs her own home-based business and she rarely buys a new dress, paints her house, upgrades her car, or even goes out to dinner – but she's one of the most abundant people I know because she's continually investing in herself. Walk into her office and you'll see an expensive ergonomic chair, the latest techno-gadgets, a serene set of art prints, and endlessly flickering aromatherapy candles.

Her home office is her sanctuary because it's there where she feels the most accomplished, creative, grateful, excited, useful, and proud. Every cent she makes goes back into marketing her business, revamping her website, fine-tuning her services, or crafting her brand. While her home décor is threadbare and dated, she continually updates and modernizes her work environment, output, and philosophy about her home business.

Rarely does she complain about being overworked because, as she points out, "when you love what you do it's never work." She literally invests in herself – her health, her welfare, her well-being, and her passion. The dividends she receives may not be immediately tangible – no fancy car or ostentatious mansion or glittering jewels or wall full of awards – but the true abundance of her life is reflected in her beaming smile, straight posture, and positive attitude.

Staying Charming With Less

So, you might be saying that all of this is well and good, but what if the bank account really is so puny that it's hard to muster

Creating Wealth in a Turbulent Economy by Tim Grizzle

Make Money, Not Excuses: Wake Up, Take Charge, and Overcome Your Financial Fears Forever by Jean Chatzky (Three Rivers Press).

On My Own Two Feet: A Modern Girl's Guide to Personal Finance by Manisha Thakor and Sharon Kedar (Adams Business).

The Secret of Shelter Island: Money and What Matters by Alexander Green (Wiley).

up a smile, lend a helping hand, or comport yourself with style and grace?

Bad economic times often lead to bad manners as people let their reduced circumstances affect their attitudes. Pressures at home mount as the bank account shrinks and the bills pile up, turning finances into a pressure cooker that can often melt the CHARM right off our backs. To me, it almost looks like the first thing to go is the very civility that makes a woman special, enticing, and CHARMing.

I know it's tough to be CHARMing when you don't know where your next rent or mortgage payment is coming from, but it's just such a time that requires your best foot forward.

Princess Julia's
CHARM Tip #7

Think about how your parents handled money when you were growing up and how that has influenced your approach to money. Were they savers and scrimpers and that has led you to be extra conservative with money, or maybe you've done a 180 and become a big spender. Or, maybe you watched them squander their hard-earned dollars as if they weren't hard-earned at all and so you grew up thinking money grows on trees, or you vowed to be more careful when you got old enough to bring in your own paychecks. Whatever the lessons learned with your parents as money models, think about which habits you may need to un-learn and which ones you could benefit from copying more.

CHARM will make you the standout candidate for the job or will be the confidence-builder to help you get a new client or even a new mate. The woman who remains unruffled in the tough times thrives, and what she needs comes to her through that age-old law of attraction.

Riding Out Negativity

Remember that CHARM is not just a way to look or act on occasion but a way of life. It is a way of thinking positively in negative circumstances, not just because we're looking at life through rose-colored glasses or even ignoring the obvious, but because we inherently recognize that "going negative" isn't going to help a thing.

Will snapping at your husband make his paychecks – or yours – any bigger? Will complaining to your friends improve any of your financial problems? Being negative creates negativity and being positive breeds positivity. CHARM is about assessing every situation – good or bad – and figuring out how to make it better through those things you can control.

Okay, so you *can't* control when a recession will end or whether your employer will decide to have big lay-offs, but you can control your reaction and your decision to make the situation better or worse. Remember that charm isn't just about you but about others as well. We are all in this together, and chances are, if you've got it bad someone else has it worse.

Have you ever caught yourself complaining about life's little inconveniences – how you can't take that summer trip you were planning or afford to put in the pool just yet – only to find out that the person you're talking to has it much, much worse? Think of what others are going through and use your CHARM to be part of the solution, not just to make more problems.

Not All Tough Times Are Created Equal

CHARM is about gratitude – being thankful for what we have and focusing on our abundance rather than what we lack. If you dwell on all that you've lost in a bad economy or a business deal gone sour, how hard is it going to be for you to put on a brave face and CHARM yourself out of that blue funk?

Put things into perspective. Your house may not be worth what it was in past years, but look on the bright side: is it still worth more than it was when you first bought it? No? Well, then look on the bright side that you still have a house while others have lost theirs!

And while the credit crunch may put a crimp in your spending, think how much you're learning about how to use cash instead of credit. Use the lean times to prepare for times of more abundance. Cut up your credit cards and create a plan for becoming debt free as soon as your budget allows. Rely more on what you have and less on credit, and your life will become more abundant with each purchase you don't make.

Emphasize what you need, not what you want, or think you want.

Gratitude is a matter of perspective. Even in bad times we can find the good if we simply take stock of our blessings and see things for what they are instead of what we want them to be.

Twenty Reasons Why I'm Grateful

Gratitude is a huge part of how bad things are or even how long it's going to take before they're good again, and so I'm constantly reminding myself how good I have it, even if things aren't quite so bright this quarter or sales are starting to slump. Remember, I may be a princess, but I'm a working princess, so as the rest of the economy goes, so go I. But still I have so much to be thankful for, and here I've gathered twenty reasons why I'm grateful:

1. I enjoy good health
2. My family is happy
3. They're healthy, too
4. I have plenty of friends
5. I enjoy my community service projects
6. I don't have too far to travel to work each day
7. My company is doing well
8. I haven't had to lay anybody off
9. My closet is full
10. So is my fridge
11. The roof doesn't leak
12. The car still runs
13. My taxes are paid
14. My head doesn't ache
15. My feet don't, either
16. I look forward to getting up every morning
17. I'm content when I go to sleep every night
18. I love what I do
19. I like who I work with
20. Every day is different

It's all about perspective. Instead of focusing on the negatives, it's so easy to focus on the positives – at least once you get in the habit of doing so.

Less Is More

Can you really be CHARMing in these trying times? Can you still lead a life of style and elegance, looking beautiful on the outside, while also remaining confident and altruistic and thus being beautiful on the inside?

The answer is a resounding "yes," if you'll just try to get by with a little less. There are dozens, if not hundreds, of ways to strip down your budget while piling on the CHARM. The next section lists some of those.

Princess Julia's Quick Tips for CHARM on the Cheap

✳ Put Your Beauty Regimen on a Budget

Looking good is part of feeling good, but not at the expense of the mortgage, your grocery bill, or the kids' braces! Figure out ways to do more with less in the area of beauty, such as coloring your hair at home or doing your own nails.

✳ Use the Replacement Rule

The replacement rule helps you add value to your weekly must-haves. If there are certain things you simply can't do without, replace them for things you can avoid. For instance, swap your Monday through Friday mocha latte for nails and a facial on Saturday. I'm sure if you look hard enough – or even just a little more carefully than you used to – you can find plenty of things to swap out each week until you're feeling more financially confident.

❋ Use Your Brains and Barter

When you work together, things always seem to be much easier. For instance, do you really need a professional caterer for your daughter's wedding or can four friends jump in to help – and make it fun in the process?

❋ Get "Used" to Buying Used

In most every city there's one really high-end secondhand store. The secret to being more CHARMing on less is to go often and spot quality as opposed to quantity. With practice, you'll get to know what's worth it and what isn't, and even when to go to beat the crowds and get there first!

❋ See Opportunity Where Others See Sacrifice

If your grocery bill is getting higher and higher and eating out is becoming more of a luxury– change your eating habits. Take the opportunity to switch to a healthy diet. Salads, fish, and chicken, for example, usually cost less than steak. The less processed, the healthier the foods- and less expesive. So if you take the time to make simple meals at home, you will be investing in your health and in your bank account. Remember that eating better doesn't always mean spending more, and that spending less doesn't always equate to sacrificing quality.

✳ Accept Financial Limitations with Grace

The women of World War II cut flour and sugar from their menus in support of the war effort and took up jobs to help support the family. Rosie the Riveter was plenty CHARMing!

✳ Make Saving Fun for the Whole Family

Don't be CHARMing alone. Include your family or roommates in your efforts to budget wisely and encourage them to act creatively to trim the expenses. Make it a family contest to see who can create the cheapest but healthiest menu for dinner, then shop together. Make one night each week a "refrigerator raid" and come up with creative family recipes using only what's in the fridge and pantry. Believe it or not, you could just make this country's financial crisis a learning – and bonding – experience for the whole family.

Being CHARMing with Less is Not for Sissies

The true test of CHARM isn't just being polite, kind, or available when it's convenient for you, but being all those things even when it isn't convenient for you, even when *you* need someone to be polite, kind, and available for *you*, and even when things look bleak on your end as well.

Change will come; that much is certain. Financial bubbles and bursts are cyclical, but CHARM isn't. When you feel CHARMing down to your core, you can always find a way to make the bad times good and the good times better. See this crossroads as a turning point in your financial future. Stop

To be greedy is to put things – money, possessions, objects, toys, homes, properties – above the only thing that really matters: people. It is impossible to be charming and greedy at the same time. Greed may not be the root of "all" evil, but it certainly short-circuits our efforts at CHARM. When we are greedy we are selfish; we want what we want, when we want it, as soon as we want it – and usually at all costs. We don't think of others and, thus, can't be CHARMing because to CHARM is to include others in our lives in a positive manner. Greed is all negative, all the time, to all people – except the greedy. So greed is high on my list of all-time, CHARM-killing pet peeves; and it should be high on your list as well!

relying on credit, quick fixes, and broken promises and rely more on cold, hard cash and what you know and trust to work for you.

We've all been guilty of spending and foolishly borrowing too much and not thinking for ourselves quite enough. As you rely on CHARM to get you through the trying times you've been through and that still may lie ahead, take comfort in the fact that you are not alone. Together, we can all pull through this, and I don't see any reason why we can't all be CHARMing while we do!

Parting Words About Abundance and Altruism

I hope by now you get that abundance does not equal money, riches, or a secure financial future, and that a lack of money does not mean you cannot be CHARMing and altruistic. Some of the most abundant people I know have the least of all, and yet they are blessed with lives that are fulfilling and absolutely CHARMing in their sincerity and security.

This has been a special chapter for me to write because charm and abundance do go hand in hand. It's easy to fall back into our default definitions of CHARM: manners, politeness, grace, and style. But we also have to remember the bigger picture and how CHARM radiates throughout not just our lives but those of our family, friends, neighbors, colleagues, bosses, and acquaintances – even total strangers.

Abundance is an attitude, not a possession. Like CHARM, abundance is something that radiates from our core and increases with use.

In the final analysis, then, what *is* abundance? When we feel full of accomplishment and pride in a job well done, that is abundance. When we look at a dinner table surrounded by smiling faces, that is abundance, no matter how simple the meal on that table might be. When we put our heads on our pillows at night and fall asleep without a troubled conscience, that is abundance.

Look in the mirror now, smile, and reflect on this chapter. Chances are, if you've been listening at all, you'll see abundance staring back!

C
H
A
R
M

$\mathcal{R}$omance is CHARMing

Romance is CHARMing

"One day you will ask me which is more important, my life or yours? I will say mine and you will walk away not knowing that you are my life."

Khalil Gibran

Like Manners, the idea of courtly love dates back to medieval times. Modern Love has rendered Romance obsolete. That is, Romance with capital R, where every phase of a relationship is carefully coaxed to its fullest expression and we allow ourselves enough time to reach the ultimate decision: keeper, friend, or neither! Too many unfortunate lovers have rushed through the process and mistaken Sex for Romance, and in the process the better part of the loving relationship has suffered.

To invite Romance into a CHARMed life requires the same diligence and attention to detail as keeping Romance in your life. Confidence is never more important than when dealing with this issue: you have to be yourself, love yourself and treat yourself with respect before you can invite others into your heart and into your life./share your life. If you are going through tough times, as we all do now and again, you may yearn for an easy way out – and let the wrong person in. And that's a recipe for disaster.

Of the five elements of CHARM, Romance is the most artful- and the most heartful – as revealed in the mystery of a carefully crafted love letter (as seen on my website), the fascinating attention to detail during a date, and the adventure of discovering everything there is to know about that special someone.

Armour may have long since gone out of fashion, but Romance will always be at the heart of the CHARMing woman.

Chapter 8

Princess Julia on the Laws of Attraction

"The most exciting, challenging and significant relationship of all is the one you have with yourself. And if you can find someone to love the you [that] you love, well, that's just fabulous."
Carrie, from Sex & the City

My grandparents had an arranged marriage back in Hungary. My grandmother was from a prominent family close to the ruling Karoly family, and she had been groomed from birth to marry my grandfather Karoly. As a young adult, she didn't love him. She was in love with someone else, someone she was not permitted to marry. Decades later, my grandparents were very much in love, and had been since the birth of their first child. This may not be your idea of how you want to find your life's mate and fall in love, but it worked for them in the long run.

Much has been said, written, and sung about love, and I don't claim to have the last word on it – or the first – but what I have learned from experience is that love can creep up on you in all kinds of ways and when you least expect it. And, I've learned that true happiness can only come from within ourselves.

First, Break All the Rules!

Now, I may be from the South but I am *not* one of those Southern women who prescribe to "The Rules," "The List," "The One," or even "The Plan" for tricking a man into loving you until death you do part. But let's get real: Putting on a little makeup and pretending to like Monday Night Football – if only to get the clicker back for the rest of the week – isn't so much tricking your man as lulling him into a more receptive state. And that?

That I'm all for!

I live by one very simple rule when it comes to dating: Break all the rules. After all, rules were meant to be broken and nowhere is that truism more truthful than when it comes to

Princess Julia's
CHARM Tip #8

Don't let not having a mate get you down on life and make you un-CHARMing. Give yourself the love you deserve, not by waiting for someone else to hand it to you on a silver platter, but by pampering and treating yourself. Bring flowers home for no special occasion. This might feel a little silly, but treating yourself with respect brings a confidence boost – and a bit of sunshine via fresh flowers you'll bring into your life is not at all silly.

dating. If *Cosmo* tells you to do one thing, consider doing the other; if a girlfriend insists such and such worked on so and so, consider doing the opposite.

Think about it: if every woman on the block is trying the same trick, technique, or tactic they just learned in this month's women's magazine, don't you think the men down at the club are going to get a little bored if you saunter up doing the exact same thing? So you can easily stand out by simply doing what everyone else isn't doing, which usually means simply being yourself.

Being yourself is the antidote to all those other rules. It makes them seem sophomoric, senseless, and downright silly. I've never understood those women who make dating a game, putting on airs, wearing clothes that aren't their style, proclaiming to like things they've never enjoyed before and laughing at jokes that aren't funny – in short, being anything but themselves – and then wind up complaining when the man they snagged doesn't like them for who they really are.

Well, he never knew you for who you really were in the first place. Why? Because you never let him see the real you; all he saw was the fake you, the one playing games and pretending to be someone else. Now what kind of foundation is that to start a relationship on? Where do you go from there?

I'll tell you where: nowhere. You either have to start all over, showing him the real you and hoping he likes it, or give up altogether because you weren't being honest with each other. So why not cut out the charade and get down to brass tacks from the get go? I'm not saying show up to your first date in curlers, house dress, and slippers – which you should never be seen in anyway – but be yourself.

If you don't like foreign films, don't agree to go to a French film fest as your first date. And if you do, just to see if you'll like it or because he's really, really convincing, then compromise; request that you get to pick where you go for the second date. If he agrees, you've probably got a flexible man that you can work with. If not, well, that's why it's called dating, not marriage!

A (Non) Rule: The Rule of Natural Selection

I have a friend – we'll call her April – who is, has been, and is likely always to be the worst dater on the planet; that's because she never feels comfortable in the driver's seat. She doesn't go out on dates; she waits for men to come to her. Not because she's selective or choosy, but because deep down I know she feels insecure and unworthy about going out and picking a man for herself.

Some women see the whole world as a singles club; April sees the same three or four settings every day. She's got her workplace, her gym, her hair salon, and her front doorstep, so basically her dating pool is all shallow end, all the time. Unless somebody new shows up at work, she's stuck with the same twenty or thirty guys she's already decided not to date.

Okay, sure, the gym has plenty of fresh blood sauntering in every few months, but either she feels too old and fussy for the young hunks or the old crows aren't interested in anything but fresh meat. And the hair salon? Well, not the best place to meet men. So, basically, unless a hunky new UPS man shows up at her door with a package, she's out of luck.

As a result, April is always suffering through mediocre relationships that leave her apologetic, disappointed, and disillusioned. Currently she's living with a man who hasn't worked since their first date. While most of us would be on this guy's case like ants on a leftover piece of red velvet cake, she's just so happy to have a man around that it's more than acceptable for him to lie around while she's out bringing home the bacon.

While she was complaining about her bills the other day I asked her, "April, when was the last time you actively went out and looked for a responsible, hard working and pleasant man to date?"

She frowned and said, "I got spoiled in high school; there was always a new guy to date and they were all there in the halls, just ripe for the picking. Where do you go to find a quality guy once you graduate?" I didn't have an easy answer for her then - so now I always have answers to many questions like that on my website -, but to myself I thought, "Well, anyplace is better than your own front door."

On the opposite end of the spectrum, my friend "Katie" is so choosy about who she dates she rarely goes out. Katie is the kind of girl who doesn't just live by The Rules; she's made some of her own. Like her "shoe rule," which states the man must wear expensive shoes or he's not worth dating; period, no exceptions. Other similar rules include the "watch rule," the "car rule" and, well, you get the picture.

Princess Julia's Favorite Books on Romance

Perfect Love, Imperfect Relationships by John Welwood (Trumpeter).

The Five Love Languages: How to Express Heartfelt Commitment to Your Mate by Gary Chapman (Northfield Publishing).

Emotions Revealed, Second Edition: Recognizing Faces and Feelings to Improve Communication and Emotional Life by Paul Ekman (Holt).

Getting the Love You Want: A Guide for Couples, 20ᵗʰ Anniversary Edition by Harville Hendrix (Holt).

How to Talk to Anyone: 92 Little Tricks for Big Success in Relationships by Leil Lowndes (McGraw-Hill).

Keeping the Love You Find: A Guide for Singles by Harville Hendrix. Holt.

The Seven Principles for Making Marriage Work: A Practical Guide from the Country's Foremost Relationship Expert by John M. Gottman and Nan Silver (Three Rivers Press).

Stop Wondering If You'll Ever Meet Him: A Revolutionary Approach for Putting the Date Back into Dating by Ryan Browning Cassaday and Jessica Cassaday (Hay House).

Women Who Love Sex: Ordinary Women Describe Their Paths to Pleasure, Intimacy, and Ecstasy by Gina Ogden (Trumpeter).

Since so few guys can abide by her many rules, she often spends nights and weekends alone, complaining about the lack of "appropriate" guys on the market. Now, I'm the last one to tell someone to lower their standards – just look at April – but some standards are not only impossible to meet, they're impractical when it comes to finding a good, quality man in the first place.

For instance, I know many intelligent, funny, gainfully-employed, handsome quality guys who couldn't care less about the shoes they wear, what time it is – let alone what brand of watch they buy – or what car they drive. By Katie's "rules," these guys are ineligible bachelors; to me, they're Bachelors of the Year.

The Exception to the Rule: You Rule!

So what is it about dating that forces us to opposite ends of the spectrum? Why are there so many women who have absolutely NO standards – I'm talking *zero* – when it comes to dating and those who have such high standards – I'm talking *hero* – that no one man can actually meet them?

Perhaps it's because so many of us have been burned by dating in the past that we tend to have one of two severe reactions once we're of a certain age: either we (a) give up and date anybody and everybody, figuring it's never going to get any better or (b) build a wall around ourselves, secretly hoping a knight in shining armor might one day penetrate our fortress of gloom and doom.

When we are jealous, it has nothing to do with the person we envy and everything to do with ourselves. What is it about us that makes us jealous of those who, on the surface at least, have it better than we do? And do they, really? You never know how happy or unhappy someone is, of how well they are really doing. Appearances are deceiving. Jealousy usually arises out of superficial judgements anyway. But it makes us question who we are, what we do, where we come from, where we live, and, frankly, why we're here. And anything that shakes us to our foundations like this, and in such a negative way, is bad for us, bad for hope, bad for courage – bad for CHARM.

Get rid of your jealousy; you are who you're supposed to be, where you're supposed to be, and, I hope, doing what you love. What could be more fulfilling than that? Be proud of who you are because, trust me, when we are proud, we are CHARMing.

For me, absolutes are rarely the answer. I tend to fall somewhere happily in the middle ground. My standards are high, but not unreasonably so. I enjoy nice watches myself, but what good is the watch on a man's wrist when the look on his face is a permanent scowl. My preference is for a good man with a wide smile, an easy laugh, and a tender heart. As Chris Noth's character, "Big," once said in *Sex & the City*, "*After a while, you just want to be with the one that makes you laugh.*"

More importantly, you've got to be comfortable in your own skin before you can ever feel comfortable on a blind date, first date, third date, or 25th wedding anniversary. For me, dating is less about looking for the right man and more about looking for the right fit. Oftentimes, the wrong man is the right man, if you know what I mean.

Some of the happiest couples I know are exact opposites of each other. She didn't find Mr. Right so much as she found Mr. Right For Her. She is outgoing and he is shy. He is irresponsible and she is respectably buttoned-up. She is tall, he is short. She is thin, he is fat. And yet it works. Why? Because it works for them.

Forget the rules, forget what your friends say, and absolutely, 100% forget what your mama told you back on the farm! At the end of the day, dating is a lot like shopping for the right car. Understandably, it's exhausting, absolutely you don't want to do it for the rest of your life, but it's 100% essential to finding the right fit for you. People are so independent, they become demanding and set in their ways. You have to really search until you find a match *for you*. You wouldn't buy the first car you drive off the lot, would you, just because it's inconvenient to keep on looking and looking? No. You drive a few more cars, kick a few more tires, check out the upholstery, and crunch the numbers. When it's right, you know it – in cars, in homes, in jobs… in men.

In short, don't drive off the lot with a lemon just because you were too lazy to keep looking for a Rolls!

Princess Julia's
Bonus CHARM Tip

You can't wait for magic to happen in life. *Give yourself permission to make realistic dreams and set achievable goals.* This is actually the most difficult step: to clearly identify where you want to go in life, with whom you want to be, where you want to live...whatever it is you want to change in your life.

Thinking about your dreams and goals won't make them come true. You have to be in a calm, positive mindset to make a plan, then to identify and harness your resources: your time, your social network, your skills, your family.

The next step is to break down your big goals into small, achievable tasks that you can accomplish a little at a time, whether one task per day, per week or per month. Remember to reward yourself every time you accomplish a landmark: a facial, a sauna, new exercise shoes.

Above all, have fun, rejoice in each small success, regroup and rethink a failure, and head onward with a smile! The journey is the most important part! Make a CHARMing road for yourself.

Parting Words about Romance

As always, I hope I've taken some of the mystique out of this topic. Dating is what you make of it. If you're the kind to over dramatize everything, from a quick trip to the grocery store to a flat tire to a broken nail to a run in your stocking, well, I imagine dating is going to be your idea of Oscar-worthy drama every night of the week.

But if you take the drama out of the equation and don't treat every date as your last-ever chance to find Mr. Right, not only will things go a lot easier for you in the long run but you might actually have some fun!

I love it when I hear that one of my friends is going on a date. What fun! What a great opportunity to try a new restaurant, meet a new fella, take in a new show or try a new adventure.

Dating doesn't have to be this whole rigorous, endless conveyor belt of frustrating experiences, excuses and lukewarm meals spent engaging in equally tepid conversation. Dating is an opportunity; you never know when Mr. Right is going to be sitting there, right beside you. And you may even overlook him if you treat dating like a chore.

C
H
A
R
Manners are CHARMing

Manners are CHARMing

"Liberty cannot be preserved, if the manners of the people are corrupted."
                                        Algernon Sidney

We face today a general lack of respect for what has been passed down from generation to generation regarding what it means to be polite, proper and refined. When it comes to setting a standard for human behavior, the concept of Manners seems archaic to the point that respect, care and consideration appear outdated.

People are so self-centered and single-minded in their quest for getting ahead in life, they run roughshod over family, friends and co-workers in order to get "there." It's all about me-me-me, my turn. When– and if– they reach their goal it becomes a soul-less place without friends, with no one to share its joys. The perfect plot for some inane reality TV show, but a poor substitute for reality, don't you think?

This book is designed to give you a roadmap to prevent this trap, and this section is divided into chapters: Social, Business, Travel and most importantly, Family Etiquette.

Yet I see a glimmer of hope when I realize that there are women like you who are still interested in becoming CHARMingly educated about Manners, despite a popular culture bombarding us with endless examples of crass, rude and offensive behavior.

After all, books selling millions of copies have been written on the subject, advice columnists answer questions of its applications in daily newspapers across the country, and entire schools have been dedicated solely to the purpose of preserving Manners.

So far we've seen that a Confident woman uses her Hallmarks to nurture Romance in her life while still finding time for Altruism- all of which are empowered by the proper Manners.

Although Etiquette may change with time, location, social stratum and occasion, one thing remains constant: socially proper behavior is never out of style.

Chapter 9

Princess Julia on Social Etiquette

"Manners easily and rapidly mature into morals."
Horace Mann

Remember the scene in the movie *The Princess Diaries* when Julie Andrews, playing the queen, calls Anne Hathaway as a freshly hatched princess into the palace drawing room for a series of lessons on how to comport like a princess? In a kind of royal boot camp, the ugly duckling was transformed into a swan at the hands of her wise and regal grandmother.

Well, I'm a graduate of that same boot camp, only mine wasn't quite so hurried and pressured, and the final exam wasn't so tough, because I was not about to take over the throne of a country. My grandmother just wanted me to carry on the proper behavior and customs that came with my royal lineage, even if my life was destined to be much more of a commoner than of a queen.

When I was a little girl, my grandmother would sit me in her lap and brush my long hair for hours on end, speaking to me in Hungarian. I understood very little of what she said, but my father would come in and translate from time to time so that I could understand her valuable lessons. She taught me everything from the importance of sitting up straight and keeping my elbows off the table, to being always nicely dressed with hair done, to treating people politely and with respect.

And, my grandmother wasn't just talk. She walked the talk, always careful about her appearance, rarely going out in public without perfectly clean, pressed, and starched clothes, her hair carefully coiffed, and when in church, always a veil and gloves. But the lesson I learned most from her was that where your elbows go and whether your hands have gloves on is only a tiny part of good manners. She taught me that respect, courtesy, saying please and thank you, enduring hardships with dignity and hard work —no complaining, just doing! – and caring for others are what good manners are really all about.

Why Manners Matter

When was the last time you pulled out your copy of *Emily Post's Etiquette*? How about any of the good books on etiquette by "Miss Manners" (Judith Martin) or "Ms. Demeanor" (Mary Mitchell)? Been a while since you've thumbed through the pages of these manners missives? Wait, what's that you say? You don't even own any these books? And you haven't even checked them out of the library? Oh, my! You're making me clutch my pearls, and that is always a sign I'm not too happy. Okay, I won't give you a lecture here, but let me tell you that these are must-reads.

This little book of mine on CHARM can only scratch the surface of the huge topic of etiquette. From knowing which fork to use first from a formal place setting, to the art of writing a thank you note when you really didn't like the gift (more on that on my website!), to when you should or shouldn't fight your business lunch companion for the check after a restaurant meal, the topic of etiquette requires almost encyclopedic writing to do a thorough job of coverage.

That doesn't mean that a crash course, manners boot camp isn't possible, though. So, strap on your boots (or your ballet flats, spectator pumps, or running shoes!) and let's take a walk on the wild side of proper behavior with some highlights of the biggest DOs and DON'Ts of social and business etiquette.

What Social Etiquette Is

More than sixty years ago, Emily Post began helping people mind their manners with her book *Etiquette*, now written and updated each year by her great-granddaughter Peggy Post and now in its 17th Edition, as of this writing. The subject is as important today as it was 60 years ago, especially since children are being raised by overworked single parents, who don't have the time to cover all the bases when it comes to covering this kind of "detail" in a young adult's education. Emily Post founded her etiquette advice on three basic principles, which still hold true today as the cornerstones of proper behavior:

✳ Respect
This means recognizing that every human being has value, regardless of background, socioeconomic status, race, creed, age, and so forth. Respect means treating everyone on

an equal basis, whether you're dealing with the CEO of a major corporation or a ditch digger.

And, guess what? It means having self-respect, too! We devotées of CHARM know all about that, don't we?! We believe that you can't respect others if you don't feel that way about yourself first. So, there you have it: As I've been saying, making the world a more beautiful place starts with you, and your beauty starts from the inside out. Respect yourself so that you can respect others, and so that the respect will continue to spread to everyone.

✳ Consideration

Okay, so you recognize the value in all other humans, but do you act on that recognition? Do you act with thoughtfulness and kindness? This is the other cornerstone of etiquette – thinking before you act, speak, react, considering how what you do or say will affect others. Etiquette is about not being selfish. It's about behaving in a way that will not offend, inconvenience, insult, annoy, or hurt the feelings of others.

✳ Honesty

My grandmother helped me realize that ethics and etiquette are interwined. Good manners should come from sincerity, not just going through the motions of following etiquette rules that we don't believe in. You write a thank-you note not just because it's expected– as a sign of respect for the other person's feelings and intentions– but because you really want to express your appreciation. That is etiquette. It's honesty we express in everything we do.

What Social Etiquette Is Not

I also learned from my grandmother what etiquette is *not*. Misconceptions of etiquette abound. No, it's not just about knowing the fish fork from the dessert fork or how to fold a handkerchief. It's about living with grace and graciousness that fits with modern-day situations and circumstances.

According to Peggy Post, there are four main things that etiquette is not:

1. A set of rigid rules.

2. Something only for the wealthy or well-born.

3. A thing of the past.

4. Snobbishness.

Good manners are for everyone and are easy for everyone to implement. Etiquette "rules" are not so much rules as they are flexible guidelines for living, whether you live in a mansion or a humble little apartment. They are not about being born a snob or becoming a snob. They are not designed to make us feel superior but, in fact, to make us more equal to everyone. They are more needed today than ever. Even though life in general is more casual than in past eras (how often do you go to a restaurant where jacket and tie is still required for a man?), the basic principles of respectful, considerate behavior are still very much in style.

> *"Good manners will open doors that the best education cannot."*
>
> Clarence Thomas

When you are wrong – yes, it *will* happen sometimes! – always own up to your mistakes or misunderstandings by acknowledging them and apologizing.

Smiling at a passerby or at someone you're standing near in a queue or sitting near in a waiting room may seem like a gesture that doesn't mean much, but it's more than just a common courtesy. It could actually change your life! You never know who that other person is. Is this the person who has a job or business connection you've been needing? Could this person become a friend? You never know. Your smile can open the door to opportunity.

Princess Julia's Advice on CHARMing Manners

Sometimes I think we've become a gum-chomping, cell-phone blabbing, curse word-slingin' society. Where have dignity and decorum gone? I'm not saying we have to be prim and proper all the time. But we really need to get back to some basics of good behavior. Here's what I think we need to do to be CHARMing and make the world a more CHARMing place:

✳ Common Courtesies

Please. Thank you. After you. May I help you with that? Such easy things to say but not said nearly enough.

Or, how about giving up your seat to someone who looks like they could use it? Making eye contact with the person at the checkout counter (or with the customer if you are that cashier). Smiling at a passerby. Saying hello when a passerby greets you. Waving your hand in thanks when a driver lets you squeeze into their lane so you can make your turn. Holding a door for someone. Keeping the elevator door open a few seconds more no matter how much of a hurry you're in. Such easy things to do but not done nearly enough!

☀ Cell Phones

Where to begin on this one, right?! Mobile phones seem to bring out the worst in people. Cell phone etiquette is simple: Keep your conversations to yourself (we really don't want to hear it…in the grocery store, in the post office line, on a plane, anywhere), don't talk on the phone while driving, and put the phone down when someone is serving you.

☀ Voice mail

How convenient that we can leave a message for someone we're trying to reach. Hard to remember there was ever a time when a phone would just ring and ring with no answer. But, how inconvenient to come home to a string of messages that say "Hi, call me back." Not leaving a name works for people we know well. But if you're not sure your voice will be instantly recognizable, state your name. And if you really don't know the person well, state both your first and last names slowly and clearly and spell them if that seems helpful.

Also, make it easy for the person to call you back. Let them know why you're calling so that they can have an idea of what they're in for when they return the call – do they need to set aside an afternoon to get into something deep or can call you two minutes before walking into an appointment because you just need a minute of their time. And, let them know when you can be reached. Do your part to minimize phone tag by giving blocks of time you should be easily reached, or days and times, if a call-back isn't required the same day.

✳ Email

Like voice mail, email has revolutionized our lives, in many ways for the better. But, where has the CHARM gone in our communications? Email messages often lack the niceties of other forms of communication. Even if you have to be brief and to the point in an email because you're in a hurry – or maybe just because you don't like to type! – take a moment to say a quick "How are you?" or "Hope you're doing well" or "Thanks."

✳ Voice Volume

I don't know if it's the earphones so many of us wear to listen to our iPods, or the surround sound speakers on our fancy entertainment systems, but we seem to have become a hard-of-hearing society that feels the need to shout. Please start taking note of your voice level, especially when in public, and see if it needs to be dialed down a notch or two.

✳ Profanity

Cursing is lazy. Think about it. If a handful of curse words can serve multiple purposes, then you don't have to stretch to use a broader range of vocabulary. Just about everything you say can have one of your good ol' standby cuss words inserted into the blank, the blank where a more unique term could have been used. Now, I'm not saying I never utter one of these words myself. Sometimes, there's just nothing more descriptive, and more satisfying to say, than profanity to express strong emotions or to drive a point home.

But, if you've gotta do it, do it in only carefully selected circumstances around carefully selected people, and preferably only in private. My friends who have children say that they can hardly go anywhere without the kids being exposed to every bad word under the sun. So, if you must curse, be aware of who is around you and realize that they, no matter what their ages, may not want to or need to hear blue language.

❋ Smoking

I know addiction is a powerful thing, so I'm not going to lecture you on why you ought to quit smoking. You've heard it all before, and if you could you would.

If you do smoke, be extra considerate of those around you. You know that secondhand smoke is damaging, so do you really want to be putting others in harm's way? Plus, it's just plain unpleasant and invasive to non-smokers. Fortunately, increasingly strict laws in public places and work places, even in countries that have always been known as smoking cultures, are making it easier for you to have good smoking etiquette. It's getting harder and harder for you to smoke in places where it could bother others. So, this piece of advice is almost a moot point these days. But, there are still plenty of places where smoking is allowed publicly, as well as all the private homes you could smoke in. So, before lighting up in any of those spots,

Princess Julia's
Favorite Books on Social Etiquette

The Amy Vanderbilt Complete Book of Etiquette: 50th Anniversary Edition by Nancy Tuckerman and Nancy Dunnan (Doubleday).

Emily Post's Etiquette, 17th Edition, by Peggy Post (Collins Living).

The Complete Idiot's Guide to Etiquette by Mary Mitchell (Alpha).

Letitia Baldrige's New Manners for New Times: A Complete Guide to Etiquette by Letitia Baldrige (Scribner).

Miss Manners' Guide to Excruciatingly Correct Behavior, Freshly Updated by Judith Martin (W.W. Norton & Company).

Multicultural Manners: Essential Rules of Etiquette for the 21st Century by Norine Dresser (Wiley).

think twice about doing so, and if you must, ask for permission to smoke or find an isolated place to go to do it.

Minding Your Manners Over a Meal

I love to eat out! Why? It's not just the food; it's the entire experience. Much like I love the shopping more than the buying, and the accessorizing more than the dressing, eating out is about a whole lot more than food. It's about the experience!

When I was a kid, and I'm thinking this may be how it was for you as well, eating out was a treat, something we did for fun. And everyone loved it. Mom was happy she didn't have to slave over a hot stove all afternoon, dad was happy because he didn't have to hear mom complain about it, and I was happy I wouldn't have to do dishes afterward. Plus, I got to dress up!

Since then, not much has changed, only now I get excited all over again. No cooking, no complaining, and still no dishes. What's not to like? To me, dining out is a little like going on vacation – without the airfare. If I'm in the mood for something exotic, I can try the little Indian place around the corner or the Thai spot downtown. If I'm in need of comfort food, there are great Italian and Southern cookin' restaurants within a few minutes of home.

I can walk into a restaurant and have an instant mood swing, for the better. Sometimes even knowing I'm going to be going out to dinner can improve my mood by a good 180-degrees, and it still has nothing to do with what I put in my mouth. For me, the charm of dining out is literally the CHARM of dining out!

So, what's the problem? Where does etiquette come in? Well, unfortunately, the CHARM of dining out gets lost when my fellow restaurant patrons aren't practicing the good principles of CHARM. Some people are better behaved when they go out to eat. Families seem to get along better, blind dates go smoother, old friends seem even friendlier, and even enemies tend to warm up when you're sitting across from them in a restaurant.

CHARM should come easily when you're dining out. But what about those who aren't so CHARMing?

While writing this book, I was staying in a hotel in Savannah, Georgia to work with my editor. Savannah's a gentile place where you'd expect most everyone to have nice manners, but the lady sitting at the table across the dining room from us during breakfast must not have been a local! We heard a clanging sound and both turned around to see what was going on. We expected to see a bored child banging a fork and knife on a plate. Much to our surprise, the sound was coming from a grown woman eating her eggs and grits. With fork in one hand and knife in the other, she had a rhythmic beat going like drumsticks on a cymbal. This wasn't just a one time, accidental slip of the silverware that caused a little clanging sound. This was a complete disregard for the peaceful environment of the breakfast room and for her fellow patrons. She was not only being rude, she was being selfish. She could have used an etiquette boot camp!

Princess Julia's Advice on CHARMing Restaurant Manners

Following these simple guidelines will help you keep from embarrassing yourself or violating any of the rules of the road for restaurants. You'll be on your way to being a CHARMING dining companion.

- Be polite at all times to everyone who serves you, from the maitre d' or hostess to the servers and bussers.

Princess Julia's
Pet Peeve #9: Loudness

I don't get how this generation thinks that turning up the volume on drivel makes it anymore interesting! What's worse, the rest of us are catching the "volume virus" and out-shouting the young folks just to be heard. If we've learned anything so far in this book, it's that CHARM is about being low-key, under the radar, consistently, effortlessly and quietly CHARMing, day in, day out, not calling attention to ourselves and shouting at the top of our lungs, "Look how charming we are! Look, LOOK at me being CHARMing!" CHARM is a lot like money, style, or class; people know it when they see it, so the last thing you have to do is shout it to the rooftops. So leave loudness at home and avoid those who engage in it; it's hard to be charming when you're standing next to a loudmouth!

- Put your napkin in your lap as soon as you are seated.

- Don't be difficult. If you have to have the dressing on the side of your salad, all oregano flakes removed from the pasta sauce, your carrots steamed only two minutes, not three, and, well, you get the picture, then you probably ought to just eat at home.

- Don't be loud and boisterous. If the occasion is that festive, reserve a private room or go to a restaurant that everyone expects is going to be like a three-ring circus.

• Wait for everyone at your table to be served before you dig into your food, unless they suggest you go ahead without them so that your food won't get cold.

• Chew with your mouth closed and don't crunch, smack, slurp, or otherwise let us hear or see your food once it goes from fork to mouth.

• When you're finished with your meal, don't push your plate out of your way. Just leave it where it is until someone comes to take it away. Also, your plate is not an ashtray or trashcan nor a resting place for your wadded up napkin. That stays in your lap.

• Leave a tip that is commensurate with the service you received, erring on the side of generosity.

Throughout all this, relax! Dining out is meant to be fun and a treat. And, if your dining companions aren't being so CHARMing, remember that good etiquette – CHARM – isn't about making someone else look bad (especially in front of others). It's about enjoying the company of others on equal footing. So, focus on your own good manners, and when you lead by example, others follow your lead – straight to the dinner table!

Making It Easier to be CHARMing When Dining Out

There's nothing worse than a wasted hour at lunch or a lukewarm evening dinner out. If it's a special occasion, the anticipation, the sparkling conversation, and beautiful ambience will be for naught if you get a rude waiter, or worse, a bad table mate. On a weekday work lunch, nothing is worse than slow service when you have a busy deadline to meet. When these things happen, it takes extra effort to remain CHARMing. To avoid these situations, consider these suggestions:

❋ Timing is Everything

It might sound nice to eat out every night, but it can actually become a chore if you do it mindlessly. To ensure a delightfully charming meal out, whether for breakfast, lunch, or dinner, make sure the time is right. If you're too busy, your table mate is too rushed, or it's not a good night or day for it, you won't have a good time and you'll end up wasting a perfectly good meal.

❋ Wait Til You Can Afford It

Checking the prices on everything you order can be stressful, or, even worse, skimping on a good tip because you opted for the pricier glass of wine or decadent dessert. If money is tight or even if the restaurant I want to go to is out of my price range at the moment, I'd rather wait until I can go and do it up right, but within my budget– enjoy the treat and manage it so that I can indulge in a nice bottle of wine, add dessert and, for heaven's sake, tip the server generously – than go and treat the meal like an obligation. Wouldn't you?

❋ The Hot Spot Isn't Always the Right Spot

Hot spots are great; that is, they're great after they're not so hot anymore! Until then, it's just crowded parking lots, long lines at the hostess stand, inordinate wait times, busy servers, rushed meals, high prices, and, sometimes, disappointing food.

So the minute I hear there's a new place in town, I mentally file it away for later but rarely go there until five to six months after it's opened. Maybe it's just me, but I'd rather have the meal be special than just bragging that I was there.

Chapter 10

Princess Julia on Business Etiquette

"A friendship founded on business is better than a business founded on friendship."

John D. Rockefeller

I've had something to say about business etiquette ever since the day as a young woman I discovered co-workers of mine gossiping – I mean nasty, stab-you-in-the-back gossip – about other women they worked with, women I thought they liked and respected. This was an eye-opening experience that shattered my trust in people I had looked up to and led me to wonder why people have to be so hateful sometimes.

Too many women leave the CHARM at home when they head out the door for work, but in my experience as a career woman and entrepreneur, I've learned that the exact opposite is actually the best course for a serious business woman. If it weren't for CHARM I wouldn't have a business in the first place. Part of what customers who buy my product are getting is the mystique, sophistication, style, and, yes, the CHARM that is beauty – beauty in a jar, at least. In fact, if it weren't for CHARM, I'd be out of business!

But you don't have to sell skincare products to find success through CHARM. As you know from Chapter 9 on social etiquette, good manners are about treating people with respect, consideration, and honesty. Don't you think those are pretty good practices in the business world, too, not just social settings? I thought so. So, business etiquette is not only about chewing with your mouth closed at a business dinner. It's about taking the high road to value your colleagues, customers, and bosses, and all business partners as worthwhile human beings.

Business must be conducted in a businesslike manner, but that doesn't mean you can't be CHARMing at the same time.

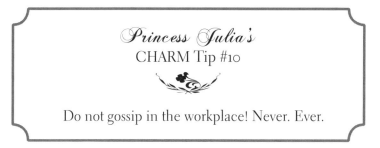

Princess Julia's
CHARM Tip #10

Do not gossip in the workplace! Never. Ever.

We Are Women, Hear Us Roar (CHARMingly)

I suppose men can be CHARMing – after all self-confidence, treating others with respect, being altruistic – those are not gender-specific qualities. But, let's face it, women have an advantage when it comes to being CHARMing. When I enter a workplace, convention center, seminar, conference, or a company, it's impossible for me to leave my femininity at the door. And it's not just because I run a cosmetics company. I'd be all lady even if I worked in a coal mine, a car wash, or on a NASCAR pit crew.

Being female is part of who I am, how I do business, and a big part of why I'm able to compete in this business in the first place. So if you're one of those women who thinks you've got to strap on a helmet and shoulder pads every time you clock in; think again. Some women feel like they have to prove themselves to be on equal footing with men in the workplace. This often comes in the form of taking on a new, work-only persona – tougher, louder, bossier, less feminine. Now, I'm all for proving oneself, but the trick comes in proving yourself on your own terms, not by trying to be "one of the boys."

My point is that either you are or you aren't; if you aren't "one of the boys," you probably never will be and that's okay. You can still get ahead in business without trying to be someone

Princess Julia's Favorite Books on Business Etiquette

Emily Post's The Etiquette Advantage in Business: Personal Skills for Professional Success, Second Edition, by Peggy Post and Peter Post (Collins Living).

The Etiquette Edge: The Unspoken Rules for Business Success by Beverly Langford (AMACOM).

Kiss, Bow, or Shake Hands: The Bestselling Guide to Doing Business in More than 60 Countries by Terri Morrison and Wayne A. Conaway (Adams Media).

Networking for Job Search and Career Success by Michelle Tullier (JIST).

else. In other words, be yourself. If you're a girly-girl, go ahead and be that way. As long as it's authentic and not put on, it should never affect your work performance or how people respond to you at work. If you're a "guy's girl," a tomboy who always fits in with the fellas, embrace that skill and live it, love it, work it!

For me to tell you to be anyone other than yourself at work is to stoop to sexism, and that's something I could never do. CHARM is all about being yourself – being the *best* self you can be.

Business Etiquette: The 10 Undeniable Rules

My nit to pick is not with women in business, but the lack of any strong or recognizable sense of business etiquette on the job, whether you're male or female. It seems this is a lost art these days, but I'm going to do my charming best to bring manners in the workplace back in vogue.

Won't you help me? Business etiquette is a trickle-down affair. In other words, it comes from the top. When the boss is rude, the managers are rude; when the managers are rude, the employees are rude and when the employees are rude – the customer suffers. And that's **never** charming! But even if you're not the boss, you can push that rock uphill and change business etiquette no matter where you are on the corporate ladder.

Let's make it our mission to bring business etiquette back to the workplace. Now, this means more than doing away with Casual Fridays; I'm talking a complete "manners overhaul" at your workplace. We'll start with the following rules of business etiquette:

✳ Manners are Non-negotiable

Manners are the mother of etiquette; they begin and end with being polite. But being polite at work is often seen as a weakness; we need to change that. What does your boss – what does any boss – want when you're at work? He or she wants one simple thing: results. Now, results are manners-blind; you can get them whether you're polite or rude. So why not get them by being polite?

✳ Class is Contagious

In all things workplace, defer regularly to class. Not upper, middle or lower class, but the tact and art of staying classy regardless of the work situation. Class is the secret weapon of the charming; it keeps us cool as cucumbers in the face of pressure and allows our brains to think clearly without being fogged up by fear, guilt, anger or envy.

✳ Kindness is Free

Just like you can get results at work by being polite, you can be a more effective employee by being kind. Ever hear the saying "You catch more flies with honey than vinegar"? I sure heard it, plenty, growing up; now I use it! I just feel like work is stressful, hard and challenging enough. Why not make it a tad better by being kind?

✳ Listening is Underrated

Listening is an often underrated business skill. When I listen, I learn; when I learn, I produce. What do I produce? *Results.* A wise person once said, "I was born with two ears and one mouth, so I should only talk one-third of the time." This is as wise a rule for business etiquette as I could come up with myself.

✳ Performance is Mandatory

Like I said earlier, results are what truly matter at work. So no matter how well you dress, how nice you are, how many Cheer Clubs and birthday parties and company picnics you organize, nothing can substitute for performance. In fact, there is nothing more polite, kind or generous than working hard, performing well and producing results.

✳ Grace is a Gift

It is such a joy and a privilege to find grace at work. How often do we come home cursing the workplace, the boss, the workload or the pile of files on our desk? Then think how easy all that would be to take with just a small amount of grace, patience, joy and appreciation as part of the mix. So what if others aren't full of grace; **you** can be, and it just may start a trend.

✳ Crankiness is Unacceptable

Work drives us all crazy from time to time, but it's bad enough without having some cranky cubicle-mate, manager or boss. What you do at work affects not just your output, but everyone around you as well. Don't inject crankiness into work; not only is it impolite, it's just plain bad for business!

✳ Politics are Polarizing

Never try to play "the game" at work; you'll always lose. Politics split offices down the middle. If you're for Bob the manager, half the office will be right behind you; but that leaves the other half, who are all getting behind Sue from Human Resources. Which side is the best to be on? Who will win? No one; splitting a workplace does nothing more than divide and conquer - and most times, divide and lose.

✳ Propositions are Preposterous

I hope I don't need to say this, but if you're looking to sleep your way to the top you'll only wind up on the bottom, no pun intended. On the bottom of the corporate ladder, the water cooler gossip parade and, of course, the lowest-of-the-low when it comes to your self-esteem.

✳ Holidays are special

Yes, I said the H-word. Holidays are a long-forgotten aspect of the workplace, whether due to budget cuts, political correctness or just plain crankiness! But from Earth Day to Thanksgiving, Halloween to Valentine's Day, what workplace couldn't benefit from a little holiday cheer?

Now, Go to W.O.R.K.

Work is a place we go to; work is a thing we do. But W.O.R.K.? That's something we believe in. To help you bring etiquette back to the workplace, I've devised this handy acronym to remind you that when it comes to being a lady, charm **never** takes a day off:

✳ W is for Women Power

Women rule. What we bring to the office is more than just facts and figures, sales and results; we bring spirit, joy, enthusiasm, grace, atmosphere, allure, sophistication, wisdom, patience and, yes, CHARM. Don't let being at work rob you of working your feminine wiles; unleash all the femininity you have and see results happen overnight!

✳ O is for On the Job

Remember that CHARM itself isn't going to get the job done. No matter what you do or say – or even how you do or say it – your boss wants results, not drama. CHARM isn't what you do at work; it's *how* you do what you do at work. Work is the cake; charm is the icing.

✳ R is for Respect the Position

Remember at all times that work is a blessing. It may not feel like it at 8:59 on a dreary Monday morning as you're still circling the parking garage looking for a space and no doubt will be doubly late for that "first thing in the morning" meeting, but to be able to work, to share your experience, your expertise and your skills is something women have been fighting for the right to do for centuries. Take advantage of that fact now and treat work like the blessing it is; charm can only follow.

✳ K is for Keep it Simple

At the end of the day, the less you think about charm in the workplace the more CHARMing you're apt to be. That's because over thinking everything – from how long to hang out at the water cooler to what to wear to Casual Fridays to how to ask out that cute new guy in Accounting – takes the emphasis off work and puts it on paranoia. Lighten up; if you got the job,

Princess Julia's
Pet Peeve #10: Laziness

There is nothing CHARMing about being lazy; sorry. Rest is one thing; relaxation another. But laziness? I won't abide for it and don't see one single reason for it. I can't wait to get up and start each new day. Even if I'm doing something unpleasant, like changing the labels on 250,000 brand new jars of skin cream, I'm eager – if not exactly happy – to do it because I know it's all part of my life's mission to work for myself, bring beauty to every woman on the planet and spread CHARM throughout the land.

When you're on a mission laziness simply isn't part of the equation. So maybe you're working at a dead-end job or only halfway through college right now; maybe you haven't worked in years and just feel "blah" when it comes to your prospects. Will sitting on the couch all day fix that? Or will taking a class, going back to school, getting to work early to produce extra reports, asking for a promotion make matters just a little bit better when this time next year rolls around? Stop thinking about yesterday, don't make excuses, and put your mind on tomorrow – it's right there, waiting for you. And I, for one, can't wait for it to get here!

they must want you around, right? So live a little and don't be afraid to be yourself.

Parting Words about Business Etiquette

At the end of the day (and, hopefully, by the end of this book), CHARM should know no bounds. There should be no distinction between work and home, home and play, Tuesday and Saturday, weddings and funerals. CHARM is not a bracelet we put on when the guests come over and then put up again as soon as they're gone. It's a part of us, a central part of our being, and work should be no different.

I'm a firm believer in taking my work home with me. Partly, that's because I own the company! But seriously, what I do is a part of who I am. I hope you feel that way, too. I hope you have the type of job where you're not afraid to be yourself, where you are respected for what you do, how you dress, what you wear but, most importantly, what you stand for.

Have you ever wondered **why** you might need a refresher course on business etiquette? Lots of times when we're happy about where we are, we're effortlessly polite, quality listeners and fabulous employees. If you're unhappy at work, try to understand why. Maybe it's not the etiquette that's so challenging, but the business you're in – or the work that you're doing.

Life is short; it's impossible to be charming when you're unhappy. If this chapter has you upset, don't shoot the messenger! Instead, think long and hard about what it is you want to do for a living and then work every day to make that happen. If it means switching jobs, getting a promotion or even going back to school, just think how CHARMing you'll be when you're finally happy at home **and** work!

Chapter 11

Princess Julia on Travel Etiquette

"If you look like your passport photo you're too ill to travel."

Joe Pasquale

Why is it that every time I make the long flight from the east coast to the west coast for some routine business I do out in Los Angeles, I end up seated next to a middle-aged man who's had two or three too many Mile-High Mojitos to drink and decides his in-flight entertainment will be to hit on me, that is, when he's not snoring and drooling on my shoulder. I guess I'm just lucky, huh? But, you know what, I try not to let it get to me. No, seriously, I try to remember that I'm lucky to be traveling on business, because I'm lucky to own a business that I love and to have a reason to go places for it. I let my attitude transport me from the seat next to a flirtatious drunk stranger to a world of gratitude and sense of adventure far, far away.

You see, "First Class" is a feeling, not a seat or row. It's an attitude, not an altitude. I don't care if you're in a plane's middle seat in the last row in coach or stuck in a closet-sized cabin with no port hole on a ship. It's all about mind over matter. Travel is an adventure to be savored. To me, few things delight like traveling someplace new, or even someplace I've been a thousand times. Even when I travel on business, I look at it as a chance to experience new sights, sounds, and people.

Unfortunately, the charm of the voyage is too often lost at sea for most voyagers. Manners, courtesy, and a positive attitude are just as likely to be lost as their luggage.

Behavior that's downright rude, obnoxious, and selfish abounds. Yes, I said selfish. Think about it: You pay good money to go on a vacation, or you have potential profits riding on a business trip, and selfish travelers come along and mess with your plans. They cut in front of you in a line, ruin your shot of the Eiffel Tower, make noise at the crack of dawn outside your hotel room door, snag the last grab-and-go sandwich as you're rushing to a plane, and, well, the list could go on and on. It's far from CHARMing behavior!

Changes in Latitude, Changes in Attitude

Jimmy Buffett got it right when he sang, "...changes in latitude, changes in attitude, nothing remains quite the same." To travel is to experience something new. It changes you, for better or worse. Why not let it change you for the better? You may not be able to control what happens to you on a trip – delayed or cancelled flights, hotel reservation mix-ups, bad food – but you can control your own attitude.

Minding your travel manners starts with minding your mind. How is your attitude affecting your travel experience, and how is it affecting the people you come in contact with when you travel? But traveling these days can be so frustrating, you say! Never fear, here are some ways you can keep your attitude CHARMing.

✳ Home Rules Apply

Wherever I go, I don't act any more formal or informal than I would when I'm at home. Would I lay out a beautiful dessert buffet when entertaining friends and then elbow them out of my way to grab the last chocolate truffle? Would I scream at the FedEx delivery guy because my package didn't arrive that day? I don't think so.

So, why do travelers get greedy, taking the last cream puff on the midnight buffet? Why do they scream at the airline ticket agent about a cancelled flight when it's not that person's fault? If we'd all simply remember that we're on vacation (or on important business travel all just trying to make a buck) travel would be a lot more CHARMing. (And they *will* make more cream puffs, people!)

✳ Don't Worry Be Happy

It should be easy to relax when you're on vacation. No fixed schedule, no working, no doing the dishes, you can stay up late and sleep in. You can lounge by the pool or bask on the beach, order room service, take a taxi, take a tour, rent a boat, shop til you drop, or take a hike. You'll be home soon enough, so wait until then to start worrying about the bills you have to pay, the garbage can you left by the curb, or whether the milk will still be fresh.

Even if you're traveling on business, you should relax. Some people use the fact that they're traveling on business –

and therefore are under more stress or have more at stake – as an excuse for bad manners. Makes me wonder how they act at work!

So, you've had meetings all morning and face a tough schedule the rest of the day, including having to go to dinner with a difficult client. You're feeling stressed and put upon. Don't take it out on your server at lunch! Fit some stress-reducers into your day, even when on business travel. Walk one block off your direct route to enjoy a lovely city park. Take a relaxing dip in the hotel pool after an evening dinner meeting. Open your eyes and really see where you are. Even if you're not in an exotic

Princess Julia's Favorite Books on Travel Etiquette

The Good Houseguest: The Etiquette of Staying in Someone's Home by Havelock James (Havelock James).

Essential Do's and Taboos: The Complete Guide to International Business and Leisure Travel by Roger E. Axtell (Wiley).

Gutsy Women: More Travel Tips and Wisdom for the Road by Marybeth Bond (Travelers' Tales).

Travel With Others Without Wishing They'd Stayed Home by Nadine Nardi Davidson (Prince Publishing).

Wanderlust and Lipstick: The Essential Guide for Women Traveling Solo by Beth Whitman (Dispatch Travels).

locale – and how much business travel for most of us really is – be conscious of the sights and sounds around you and be appreciative that you're in a new environment away from your work-a-day four walls or commuting traffic.

Join the Culture Club

World borders are growing fuzzy with so many of us doing business abroad and traveling more readily in areas foreign to us, so it's almost inevitable that you'll run up against someone who's not exactly like you on your next vacation or business trip. Whether traveling across an ocean or continent or just to a neighboring town, please be respectful of local customs and cultural sensitivities. What seems foreign, odd, funny, or even wrong to you, is second nature, maybe even sacred, to locals.

❄ CHARM is a Universal Language

Even if you don't speak the language of the country you're in, you can still communicate in a CHARMing way. Smiles translate into all languages. So does opening a door, helping someone cross a street, holding out a chair, leaving a generous tip, and being polite. Words aren't necessary with those gestures. How hard is it to start with a smile or learn just one or two words of greeting in another language? Not very, but the rewards are immeasurable. Just ask the person you end up meeting!

❄ Raise Your Cultural IQ

Find a little time before your trip to learn about the place you're going. What are the rules, laws, and customs? What are the people like? What's important to them? How do they dress and expect me to dress?

Doing your homework can keep you from being arrested for spitting in Singapore (not that you should be spitting anyway – how unCHARMing!), from photographing someone whose religious faith forbids it, or from insulting someone for cooking a meal you find disgusting but that happens to be the national delicacy.

Mind Your Ps and Qs on Planes, Trains, and Automobiles

And in hotels, airports, ships, and anywhere else your travels take you. We've all experienced it...the traveler who hogs the armrest on a plane or curses at the ticket agent for a flight delay. The kids running and screaming up and down hotel hallways or the teen-aged girls – or even worse, middle-aged! – trying to enter the Vatican in short shorts and halter tops.

If I were given a royal edict over travel etiquette, these are the ten rules I'd enforce:

1. Treat all staff – airline agents, hotel bellhops, restaurant folks, tour guides, everyone – with respect and courtesy. Most of the time, the problems aren't their fault.

2. Get your act together while standing in the airport security line, and don't wait til you get to the front to dig for your ticket and ID or take off all that jewelry.

3. Before you recline your seat on an airplane, look behind you to make sure that you're not about to crush the cover of an

open laptop or send a glass of red wine splashing into someone's lap. And, do you really need to recline that far back? Doing so can make the flight miserable for the passenger behind you.

4. If you have been known to snore or mutter in your sleep, then you may want to think twice about falling asleep on a plane if you have passengers sitting on either side of you.

5. Speaking of planes, if someone is occupying the seat in front of you, be considerate when you get up out of your own seat. So often, passengers grab hold of the seat in front of them to pull themselves upright in tight quarters. Before yanking your neighbor's seat back, figure out another way to get your body up and out of your space.

6. Arm rest sharing, or arm wrestling over arm rests? First of all, if someone is stuck in a middle seat, that person is entitled to use both arm rests. It's an unspoken rule of frequent flyers. In other cases, be considerate and take turns.

7. Whether traveling by plane, train, or bus, keep carry-on baggage to a minimum, and when putting it in overhead bins or under the seat in front of you, don't take up more space than you absolutely need. If that jacket of yours needs such tender

Princess Julia's
CHARM Tip #11

You catch more flies with honey than with vinegar. Be nice and polite to the hard-working folks in the travel industry and you might end up with perks instead of pain.

loving care and must stretch flat across an entire overhead bin to stay unwrinkled, then maybe you need to ask if a flight attendant can hang it up for you.

Princess Julia's
Pet Peeve #11: Anger

Anger isn't just one of my pet peeves; it's a sin. (Or should be!) To me, anger is dangerous; it implies some very large unsolved issues in the angry person's past. I know we all get mad from time to time, but that's not what I'm talking about here. Sometimes you can't hold your anger back and you experience a desire to fight back at the source of your discomfort or take it out on someone– you act rudely in public, devise wrathful vengeance, engage in road rage and are generally just an abusive member of society. Can you see how this could be a pet peeve, let alone the opposite of CHARMing?

Before you even blink, breathe! Take a gulp of cool water, and buy yourself some calm-down time as you try to unwind– even if you have to punch a pillow behind closed doors. Try meditating a few minutes a day in the morning– it calms the nerves and helps you think more clearly.

You simply can't be charming when you're angry because CHARM comes from a place of peace, trust, generosity and tranquility. Anger disrupts that, body, mind, and soul balance.

8. Keep it down! You, your children, anyone traveling with you – remember that you are not alone when you travel. People in that hotel room across the hall from you might be getting a rare opportunity to sleep late and really don't want to hear you screaming down the hall to your husband not to forget to pack his toothbrush as you try to get on the road at 5am.

9. Mind the noses. Be aware of strong cologne, powerful hair products, and anything else that might assault fellow passengers' olfactory senses in the close quarters of planes, trains, buses, and even car travel.

10. Finally, dress appropriately! The days of tailored suits, starched blouses, pantyhose, and pumps for travel may be gone (thank goodness – with distances between airport gates being sometimes endless, imagine how uncomfortable we'd be in high heels!), but that doesn't mean you can wear sweatpants. You are still out in public, you never know who you might meet or run into, and you need to show respect for the places you're going and the people you're interacting with. Your sweat suit and skimpy camisoles are for the privacy of your home or hotel room.

So, there you have it. Lots of ways to make the travel experience more pleasant for us all, and for yourself in turn. This whole book is about how to make the world a kinder, gentler place by being more CHARMing ourselves and spreading the CHARM to everyone we come in contact with. But, if you think about it, travel may relate to that goal more than any other topic in this book. During our travels is when we have the chance to interact with more people in more far-flung places than in our day-to-day routine in our own neighborhoods.

When we travel, we are representing our family, or our own business or the company we work for. We reflect our profession or our industry and the schools we attend (especially when wearing your school or college t-shirt or sweatshirt on a trip!). We represent our hometown or home country. We are walking ambassadors on many levels.

If each of us can remember this when we travel, and remember to exude CHARM at all times, we not only will make the folks back home proud, we will serve as role models to help make the world a more CHARMing place.

Chapter 12

Princess Julia on
Family Etiquette

*"The family. We are a strange little band of characters
trudging through life sharing diseases and toothpaste,
coveting one another's desserts, hiding shampoo,
locking each other out of our rooms, inflicting pain and
kissing to heal it in the same instant, loving, laughing,
defending, and trying to figure out the common thread
that bound us all together."*

Erma Bombeck

While working on this book, I experienced a family tragedy.
My parents were victims of a house fire. My father, sadly, died
from his burns and injuries. My mother survived but suffered
serious burns and a spine fracture. After she was released from
the hospital and rehabilitation center and was able to return
home, I began caring for her during her recovery. I've been
taking her food, doing things around the house, just generally
attending to her needs. Nothing I'm looking to earn a medal
for, just the things a daughter does for a mother in her time of
need.

Most of the time, my mother has been grateful for my
attention and assistance, but one day, the mental stress of her

condition must have tipped the scales and she turned ungrateful, demanding, even hateful. Her words felt like daggers in me. So, I disengaged for a while. I stopped coming around and let her stew in her nastiness juices. Then, I realized that I wasn't doing either of us a favor by acting that way. I felt guilty for not being there for her and worried that she needed my help and wasn't getting it. And yet, I also felt guilty for just walking away and not standing up for myself and my right to civil treatment.

So, I went back over one day and told her how her words and actions had hurt me and that I would not stand for that sort of treatment. I was stern, but in the back of my mind I knew that I was also letting it go. I had to show her that I was standing up for myself, but I knew that to find peace in my own heart and mind, I would have to say my piece and then move on and not dwell on what had happened.

My mother ended up apologizing to me on the spot, and from that moment on, has been the sweet, gracious person I know and love.

You Bring Out the ~~Best~~ Worst in Me

This is the last– but most important– chapter precisely because if there are two words that rarely go together in our modern, fast-paced, individualistic culture, they are "charm" and "family." I'm not sure why it is, but there is just something about family that brings out the worst in some people. Please understand, I love my family and I'm sure many of you love your family, too. Maybe you even get along just fine with them! But for some of you who don't relish family reunions, I want to include a chapter that applies the lessons learned throughout this book on the most difficult situations, when CHARM is in the greatest need! That means taking into consideration dysfunctional families, happy ones, separated ones, all kinds without exception. Let's face it, most families are dysfunctional to some extent, but remember what my grandmother always said: no excuses, just practice!

And, if you also factor in that I'm from a royal lineage that was not known for its display of affection-- the discipline used to train my father made him a very hard man, almost "unreacheable"–then I'm sure you can appreciate that it was not easy growing up without hugs and kisses and cuddles and other fond feelings. Maybe that sounds familiar to you, but life goes on, and this chapter is designed to help you through those tough times with the only crowd we cannot choose: family.

Family Manners Matter

So, why does the subject of family belong in this section on manners and etiquette? Isn't etiquette all about how we should behave around other people, people we don't know so well, not the people we can be ourselves around? Wrong! That's just where part of the problem lies: Because we get comfortable around our family, our sense of decorum and courtesy is often misplaced or forgotten. We can become unkind and inconsiderate, or even worse, we might spur our loved ones into being impatient or unkind with us. It's a cycle of bad behavior we have to break.

But how can we be CHARMing about a subject that's so prickly for some people? Remember, CHARM is about the total person, not just the parts you like or the situations that are easily resolved. For better or worse, family is a part of who we are and we can't be at our best unless we find a way to be CHARMing – even with our least favorite uncle who never has a kind word, or the sibling who never chips in with his/her share of family responsibilities.

Putting Perspective on Family

The first step to maintaining your good relationships with your family is to keep issues in perspective. Place the best part of the relationship top of mind. In this way we approach the problem from a positive perspective. After all, many of our issues with family are a matter of perception, not reality; the larger part of the problem sometimes exists only in our mind.

Families have become so spread out across the country that relatives frequently lose touch– and lose the emotional ties that bind. Instead of feeling joy and anticipation for reunions and holidays, I have heard many people comment on how difficult it is, how stressed it makes them feel. This negative anticipation is a foregone conclusion– they are suffering ahead of time, needlessly, with no basis in reality. That's when I bring up the issue of perception versus reality. If you find yourself in such a situation, step back from the situation and view it from a more realistic perspective, not a self-imposed one.

The first step in adopting a realistic perspective is by taking stock of your feelings. Identify your misgivings. Make a list of things that can go terribly wrong. Trace back over the course of the relationship and find the point where problems started.

Where did things begin to go wrong and what steps did you take to right them? If you take the time to chart the course of your relationship–and will be totally honest with yourself and fair to the other party–then you will eventually get to the bottom of your "issues" based on fact rather than on false perceptions that in time have turned into distorted reality.

❋ Prepare to Persevere

After you've charted the history of your relationship–and this is also a useful tool in marriage–then outline a plan of how you can improve the situation and make amends. In what ways can you make the next reunion or encounter memorable in a good way? Focus on the positive and the happy common ground you share. Avoid unpleasant ancient history. Build up a reserve of positive emotions in advance of the reunion or encounter in anticipation of the issues that may arise. We are all human, each with many flaws, so you can bet that issues will arise. What matters most is how we handle them when they do, and by this point in the lesson I expect you to remember the password: CHARM.

❋ It Takes Two to Tango, Three to Trio

If family is an issue you need to work on, call it what it is and work on it. Don't waste time dreading the reunion or stewing over any unpleasantness afterwards–that's just perpetuating old behaviors! Face the fact that part of the problem is your fault. If spending time with the in-laws is truly unpleasant, okay, we can all relate. But put the situation in perspective: when you marry someone you also marry into their family. Sooner or later, the war will be fought in your house, not theirs, and that does not make for a happy marriage. So come prepared to the next family gathering with your emotional bank account filled with an inexhaustible supply of CHARM. During the encounter, use direct and caring language at every turn, avoid personal questions while dodging questions that can lead to disagreement. Maintain a neutral position whenever others draw lines and choose sides. Be the voice of reason should disputes arise. Seek the high ground; avoid saying anything that you will regret.

You know some of the techniques already: if you feel the urge to spit out an ugly answer, quickly think of a clever response, like comics do! Or, like a politician, change the subject altogether and quickly interject a comment about a pleasant or funny common experience. Or simply ask a question of the agitator that avoids the sticky issue at hand and allows them to hold forth. Sometimes all they want is attention anyway. Let them talk.

If a relative talks your ear off it's probably because they have no one else to listen to them. How many people pay them the compliment of sharing a meaningful conversation with them? Chances are there are some lonely people in your clan. That doesn't mean a long conversation is guaranteed to be a pleasant experience, but with perspective in mind, it's much easier to navigate.

So you see, it's up to you how pleasant or unpleasant you want it to be. And that's CHARM in a nutshell: making the most of a difficult situation!

✳ Make the Most of It, Coming and Going

If you are like some people who find family gatherings unpleasant, use these tips to make them more enjoyable.

Princess Julia's
Favorite Books on Family

100 Simple Secrets of Happy Families: What Scientists Have Learned and How You Can Use It (100 Simple Secrets Series) by David Niven (HarperOne).

The Family You've Always Wanted: Five Ways You Can Make It Happen by Gary Chapman (Northfield Publishing).

How to Be an Adult in Relationships: The Five Keys to Mindful Loving by David Richo (Shambhala).

Open the Door to Better Communication with Your Teen: The Family Movie Night Prescription by David Garrison (Love & Logic Press).

Parenting With Love And Logic by Foster Cline and Jim Fay (NavaPress).

Why Can't You Read My Mind? Overcoming the 9 Toxic Thought Patterns that Get in the Way of a Loving Relationship by Jeffrey Bernstein (Da Capo Press).

Another friend of mine has to travel 210 miles or so of boring interstate to visit her mother. She has a normal and close to CHARMing relationship with her mother, but making those trips once a month gets to be taxing. Recently, my friend pulled off at an exit about halfway there and discovered a lovely little bed and breakfast with a fun gift shop and cozy café. Now, she and her husband always book a night there on the way back from visiting her mom so that the trip isn't quite so tiring. In fact, she loves the place so much she says she is almost ready to make the trips twice a month now!

Best of all, since she knows she'll soon be spending a romantic getaway at a favorite spot after the trip, she finds it much easier to be CHARMing when her mom is less than CHARMing herself– and that's what I mean about building credits into the emotional bank account.

Reasons Families Fuss and Fight - Transform Them Into Fuss and Make Up

Why is it that family can get to us while at the same time we have so much more tolerance and patience with complete strangers? Sometimes it's the baggage that exists in every family -- the secrets, feuds, betrayals, past bitterness, and close proximity of family members to our deepest, darkest secrets.

From how some friends describe it, it's like we all revert to teenagers, eager to slam the door on our folks and siblings the minute they say or do something "uncool" instead of working things out. Working on relationships is hard work. It takes determination to love and stay in love. So if you let it slide, you are making a mistake, and risking solifdifying that unresolved issue into your emotional repertoire. You want to store postive examples, not uncool ones.

Whatever the underlying reasons for a collective mis-behaving, if you're going to find CHARM in all things, you must find it with family first.

Before opening your mouth to say something less than kind to a relative, imagine that person is a new friend you've just become acquainted with. Just because you may have unresolved issues from the past does not give you license to be rude. You will find it easier to voice a courteous response if you mentally list situations where this person has helped you in the past, or was kind to someone close.

We are often kinder and more courteous to strangers than to our own family. That is less than CHARMing.

So let's see some ways we can turn the table around to our joint advantage and turn them into CHARMing family gatherings and interactions.

❊ A Wealth of Information

Families know everything about us. From who you've dated, to how much you're in debt, to that fender bender last week, to your deepest, darkest secret snack eating habits – they're privy to it all. And they not always use that dear and intimate information in a constructive manner when it comes to arguments. The flip side is, you have a common ground or foundation to build upon. A meaningful relationship has to be based upon solid ground. Use your common ground to build and strengthen your bond, not to corrode it.

❊ Photographic History

Families share pictures! They know what our hair looked like in the 80s, and they all thought it was beautiful at the time. They've got wedding photos of beautifully dressed cousins and best friends, candid snapshots from our time in the delivery room, posed family portraits when we were young and healthy, family vacations at the beach, and countless occasions. What better treasure trove to draw upon?! Use these pictures to trigger fun conversations. Laugh together– not *at* each other, *with* each other! That's a CHARMing difference. Find photos of situations all share and can be comfortable having fun with. This alone is enough to make a memorable family reunion.

❊ Pushing Buttons -- What Buttons?

Families sometimes push our buttons. Sometimes they do it just for fun, other times they don't even know they're doing it. It's up to you to take a deep breath and make a quick mental check – is this an unresolved issue on my part? If that comment -or question– is so sentive to me, do I need to look at what insecurities on my part this is pointing at? Am I supposed to be working on this issue, but instead, have let it slack – and now it shows? Whatever the dynamics, use the reactions they elicit- - your buttons– as a free consult with the shrink. Only you do the work yourself. I always remember my grandmother Julia. For her, it was not up for discussion, you had to do the work you had to do!

❊ They Can Be Physical

Sisters will cuddle and embrace. Brothers will stick up for the little sister. Aunt May kisses all the nieces and nephews because she had no children of her own. Whatever the family dynamics, many of my friends tell me that somewhere along the line, this physical closeness wears off. Some of that is "lack of practice." I have noticed that families who live in close proximity tend to be more affectionate. It is as if they reinforce the emotional and physical bond at each interaction. All I can say is, it feels wonderful when you get a strong and loving embrace. Don't deprive yourself of one. When it comes to family, be perky, cheerful and CHARMing, even under difficult circumstances, and you will be rewarded, one embrace at a time.

✳ Some of My Best Friends Share My Last Name

Like they say, "You don't choose your family." While some of us have the blessing of true and dear friends outside our family, the opposite if just as true. Just like you weed out people who you don't share a relevant bond with, it's up to you to look for the things you like in your family. They can be fun and funky, quiet and bookish, or thoughtful and considerate, just like us. They can be the source of a social network, a job interview, lend us a helping hand in difficult times.

When it Comes to Family, Listening is Golden

A colleague recently had to put his grandmother in a nursing home after she had lived independently in her own home for more than sixty years. Needless to say, it was a traumatic experience, so my friend wasn't surprised when his grandmother got upset every time he, his brother, and their mother went to visit. Things got so unpleasant that he stopped going for two weeks. Then, on a Monday, he decided to swing by and visit unannounced – and alone.

He found his grandmother in great spirits, appreciative of his visit, and eager to dig into the box of chocolates he'd picked up for her on the way there. He couldn't believe the change in her, and brought it up toward the end of his visit. "That will teach you," she winked, "to visit me one at a time. You know, my hearing's not so good and when you all start talking at once, it makes it harder for me to hear. I'm afraid I haven't been handling that very well…" It all made sense to him after she had explained it. Now he visits her one-on-one and finds the experience much more satisfying.

Princess Julia's
Pet Peeve #12: Slacker Siblings

If you have siblings and your parents need your help as they get older, be sure you pull your weight to share the responsibility of care as equally as possible with your siblings. While some of you may be geographically closer to your parents than others, and so hands-on support may not be difficult; some of you may have less income availability than others; some of you may have a larger immediate family to take care of than others; some of you may have two jobs to make ends meet –no matter what the situation, make sure you do what you can to pitch in no matter what the hurdles may be.

We all know what it's like not to be heard. Just remember your own experiences: make a mental list of things your husband or boyfriend tunes you out on, or that your mother refused to heed when you were a teenager, and so on. I'll bet you can make a pretty long list. If that is the case, it means there is at least one person at the other end who can make an even longer list directled at you! Remember, it's much easier to be CHARMing when the odds are even.

Another example is if you know your mom is going to ask what you're doing for Christmas the minute you walk in the door for Thanksgiving, make sure you're prepared to answer properly. Tell her the reasons why you can't do both holidays in one year. It's your husband's family's turn this year, you haven't been away for Christmas in years and you've already booked a room in the mountains, whatever it is you have planned. Make sure she understands that you have your husband's family to spend time with as well, and just as importantly, that you both have limited vacation time. Sometimes you need to spend time just the two of you. Tell your mom how important that is to both of you, and you don't love her any less. Needy moms can be like that. Focus on need, ladies. Be compassioante and remember the times you were needy yourself.

CHARM Begins With You

So what's the secret to being CHARMing with family? It has to start with you. You have to be the bigger family member, the better sister, the stronger daughter, the friendlier niece, or the kinder granddaughter. CHARM isn't so much about turning that frown upside down as it is turning the other cheek and being the bigger, better, kinder, more thoughtful person.

As I've said before, CHARM is contagious. The more people who experience it for themselves – through a born CHARMer like yourself – the more apt they are to receive it, own it, and spread it around. So, the more CHARMing you can be in family situations, the less offensive others are likely to be.

We all know that most family disagreements revolve around tiny, petty things – things that won't hurt us to ignore, overlook, or write off. Like the stepmother who calls your fiancé your "date" - firmly and politely correct her if the situation permits, and move on. Or make a funny comment.

A situation is what you make of it – and there's no reason you can't have a little fun while showing off a little CHARM.

Parting Words about Family

We've seen in this chapter that a family encapsulates a microcosmos of our own society. There are those members we love and are bonded for life with, there are the ones that are distant and cool, even the ones we feel we don't share the most basic emotional ties with. All in all, they are our family, and interacting with CHARM in family situations is the most prestigious manner to demonstrate that you have succedeed in applying the lessons we have learned in this book.

Use them to your advantage. Begin to see yourself as no more, no less important than anyone else in your family, and if you've felt neglected or underappreciated in the past, embolden yourself to play a stronger role from now on. Remember that confidence you learned about in the first few chapters of this book? Now's the time to let it go to work for you! When you feel good about yourself, you're in a better position to deflect the jabs and jeers and jokes that have hurt you in the past; or to lend a loving ear to the neglected cousin or older aunt.

Use your Hallmarks as talking points to demontrate to your dear Aunt May or your mom that you have listened to their lessons when you were little. Give them credit for some of your hard work-- in your heart you know you did it, but it will be a precious gift to them to know they are and were important to you.

Use Altruism to exercice the art of listening, the art of dodging loaded or tricky questions, and for making time to spend with relatives in need. Remember that we agreed that you must first focus on what you can do for those closest to you. Community service is really about helping and caring for anyone who needs you, starting with your family first.

I need not say that we will use Manners in all family gatherings, at all times.

We've discovered that CHARM doesn't grow on trees or show up in Christmas stockings. It comes from within, and the way to include "CHARM" in your family life is to cultivate your common ground and work on the ones that are not. The only way to CHARM them is to accept them, and to do that you must first accept your role as an active family member.

Afterword

There is so much going on in the world today and so much of it is tragic or unpleasant. You can't turn on the television any more without being bombarded by bad news. Some of my critics may ask, with all these crises going on in the world, why do I have no qualms about saying that I want you to go forth and be CHARMing? I can say it because to CHARM others is to care for them, to respect them, and to feel good about yourself. And to be sure, you can only make a difference one person at a time! It takes only one interaction to generate positive emotions and behavior –so this is my and your contribution to a better world, your world.

And as I said in the Introduction, you start by caring for yourself. When you have shed all the negativity that is put upon you by upbringing or peer pressure or societal values, as I talked about in the chapters about Confidence, you begin to find the real you—the chapters about Hallmarks and branding. When you do that, you begin to build an "inventory" of positive emotions. The more you practice, the more credits you put away in your heart: in Romance, in practicing good Manners, and in everyday situations. Soon you have enough "credits" in your heart to be able to spread it out in the form of compassionate interaction. Not to mention Altruism and the practice of charity, large and small. You will find that with enough credits you will be amazed to find that you are able to handle difficult situations in a more caring and even efficient way – more constructive, if you will –where before you used anger or rudeness.

Sure, table manners may seem kind of silly when so many people in this world have no food to put on a table. And, finding your signature style with the right haircut or cut of jacket may seem trivial when the fashion industry continues to turn underdeveloped nations into factory sweatshops.

I don't claim to be solving all the world's problems with the concept and practice of CHARM. But, I do know that how we treat each other is important. You know, we take certain freedoms for granted in this country, so when your representative is not doing their job, not representing you, it's a CHARMing thing to write or call that office for an explanation and be heard. That's one way to make a small contribution to influencing world problems. The politician is in the forefront, it's his job, but it's your job to be CHARMing about matters of importance to you.

Of the many ways to build and demonstrate your CHARM that I discussed in the book– and many more in my website – you will see that CHARM is not silly at all, it's part of changing the world, or, making your world more beautiful, one person at a time. So, I know that with Confidence, Hallmarks, Altruism, Romance, and Manners, we can each make our little corner of the world a more beautiful place – from the inside out.

I thank you in advance for joining me on my mission to bring CHARM back into our world, and I wish you much happiness and success in your life!

Meet me at *www.TheCharmBook.com* for ,videos and plenty of tips for a CHARMing life.

Princess Julia Karolyi

About the Author

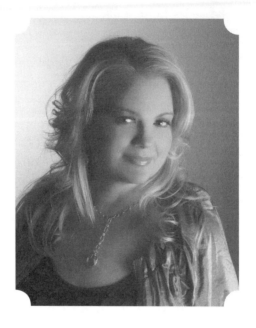

An exiled Hungarian princess and cosmetics company president, Julia Karolyi is on a crusade to make the world a kinder, gentler place. Bringing beauty, grace, and caring back into our lives, Princess Julia's mission is to take the stress and strife out of a society in turmoil.

A former rising star with beauty behemoths Revlon, Clinique, Arden, and Dior, Princess Julia became a cosmetics industry maverick by founding her company Beautage (www. Beautage.com) to deliver couture quality skincare products without the New York hype and high cost. She is currently working on line extensions to include fragrances.

Princess Julia knows, however, that true beauty comes from inside us, not from a jar. From being a cancer survivor to losing loved ones in untimely deaths, she has emerged from tragedy with a desire to spread kindness and care to all she touches.

Princess Julia appears regularly on TV and radio and speaks to groups on beauty topics and motivational strategies for living a CHARMing life.

www. TheCharmBook.com

www.Beautage.com

www.PrincessJulia.com

What the Critics Are Saying

"Finding success and happiness today in a tried-and-true secret from yesterday. After reading CHARM your perception of everyday life will change for the good, allowing you to be more comfortable and true to yourself...giving you a foundation of how to treat others."

~ Robert Hallowell
Celebrity hairstylist, The Kitchen Beautician Inc.

" Common sense advice for those who want to improve their lives – inside and out –from a woman who can help us all look better and be better than we are."

~ Lucy Morgan
Pulitzer prize winning author, St. Petersburg Times

On Beautage®:

"Julia takes the best of what she learned at Elizabeth Arden and Dior to deliver a couture-level product to the rest of us."

~ NBC, Atlanta & Company Television

"Beautage® absolutely performs like no compounded formulary I have seen and the performance of the ingredients is unfettered, powerful and dynamic. The prevention of the denaturization or breakdown of the bio-peptides in Beautage® is an exciting advance."

~ Dr. Jerry Whittemore, MD, Beverly Hills